# CONSTIPATION

## Foods, Supplements & Herbs

Isabel M. Rivero

# COPYRIGHT & CREDITS

## CONSTIPATION. Foods, Supplements & Herbs.
### Copyright ©2017, 2024 *by* Isabel M. Rivero
### All rights reserved

Cover design: Desirée Mendoza M.
Photographs by Buntysmum and Imagemo via Pixabay

This book provides general information and is not a substitute for professional medical advice. Neither the publisher nor the author shall be held liable for any damages of any kind arising from the use of this content. Readers assume full responsibility for their decisions, actions, and outcomes.

This book is intended as a reference only and should never be used as a medical manual. Its purpose is to help readers make informed decisions about their health. It is not intended to replace any treatment prescribed by a doctor.

Original title: *Estreñimiento. Alimentos y Plantas Medicinales* © 2017, Isabel M. Rivero. All Rights Reserved
© 2024 translated *by* Laura Mendoza & Sara I. Afonso

# Prologue: A Guide to Wellness

Dear Readers,

Welcome to this journey toward better health! Since I began sharing my knowledge and experience, my primary motivation has been to make a positive contribution to your lives. That's why, through these pages, I aim to offer valuable information and practical resources that can genuinely help you feel better.

In this book, every piece of advice and remedy has been thoughtfully chosen for its proven effectiveness and practicality in everyday life. You will discover not only medicinal plants, supplements, and accessible foods but also detailed medical insights into this health concern, along with additional tips and answers to the most frequently asked questions–providing you with a practical, comprehensive, and trustworthy guide.

My goal is for this work to be your valuable and practical companion–a resource where you can find tangible tools to support you on your journey toward a healthier, more fulfilling life. Knowing that this work has a positive impact brings me great joy and motivates me to keep going. While writing requires effort, time, and perseverance, the knowledge that my books make a meaningful difference in your lives is my greatest reward.

Because your experiences are my greatest source of inspiration, I would love for you to write to me and share your progress. Feel free to share your progress by writing directly to me at **isabelmriveror@gmail.com**. Your stories inspire me and truly make my efforts worthwhile.

I sincerely hope this practical guide becomes your indispensable pillar on your journey to better health and well-being. Thank you for allowing me to be part of your life. With love, Isabel.

# INTRODUCTION

On our journey towards achieving optimal health, it's crucial to recognize one fundamental truth: no single "miracle" solution –be it a medication, herb, supplement, or food–can fully resolve an illness on its own. Solely focusing on managing symptoms, while neglecting the deeper "root cause," not only delays true healing but also increases the likelihood of recurrence. Instead, addressing the underlying cause of the problem can lead to a gradual reduction in symptoms and support genuine, long-lasting recovery.

You may have experienced times when treatments or medications didn't seem to deliver the results you had hoped for. This often occurs because restoring health requires a holistic approach–one that goes beyond surface-level treatment to target the root cause of the issue. Effective healing involves more than just the right therapies; it must also encompass vital changes. A well-rounded plan should include improvements to diet (the cornerstone of cellular health), enhanced sleep quality, better stress management, and the cultivation of healthier daily lifestyle habits. Together, these elements strengthen the body's resilience, boost confidence in recovery, and reinforce its natural ability to heal.

This book takes you on a journey through this integrative approach to health and recovery. In the first chapter, we'll provide you with accessible, straightforward explanations of the main causes behind this particular illness. Additionally, we'll cover its key symptoms, variations, early warning signs, potential complications, practical advice to manage them, and the essential medical tests necessary for an accurate diagnosis. This foundation sets the stage for understanding your condition and equips you with the tools needed to address it effectively.

As the chapters unfold, you'll discover practical, evidence-based strategies designed to support your recovery. These include detailed dietary recommendations, easy-to-follow meal plans tailored to your needs, and natural approaches such as supplements and herbal remedies that support gradual, sustained improvement. The guidance provided is both flexible and adaptable, allowing you to choose what works best for your unique health journey.

For those seeking a clear roadmap, the chapter titled **"Suggested Practical Plan"** serves as a comprehensive guide. This section consolidates the most important elements of recovery into an actionable framework, while also pointing you toward additional chapters for deeper insights and tailored advice. By using this plan as your foundation, you'll gain clarity and confidence in navigating the steps toward healing.

It's worth stressing that the guidance in this book is not based on subjective opinions or anecdotal evidence. Rather, every recommendation is supported by scientific research and validated by credible studies. To further reassure you, we've included a comprehensive list of references and studies at the end of the book. This ensures you can trust the methods and feel secure when implementing these strategies into your life.

Through a blend of understanding, practical tips, and scientifically-backed solutions, this book aims to empower you as you work toward true recovery and lasting wellness.

# CONSTIPATION

Constipation is one of the most common disorders of the digestive system and, while it is sometimes underestimated, for those who experience it, it can become a persistent source of physical and emotional discomfort. It is primarily characterized by the difficulty or infrequency of bowel movements, typically defined as fewer than three movements per week. However, it is crucial to recognize that every body follows its own rhythm, and what is considered "normal" can vary greatly from person to person. The key is to pay attention to your body's signals—discomfort, changes in your regular bowel movement pattern, and a persistent sense of unease should never be ignored.

To fully understand what happens during constipation, it is helpful to first understand how the digestive system functions under normal conditions. The process begins with food intake, which travels to the stomach, where it is broken down with the assistance of gastric juices. From there, the remnants of the food move into the small intestine, where essential nutrients needed for the body's functions are absorbed. What remains from this process is then transported to the large intestine, where one of the most essential steps occurs: the formation of stool.

The large intestine, also known as the colon, plays a central role in the digestive process. Its primary function is to absorb water and electrolytes from the food residues, which not only maintains the body's hydration but also determines the proper consistency of the stool. Stool should ideally remain firm enough to allow for smooth passage, yet not so dry as to cause difficulty. At the same time, the colon performs muscular contractions known as peristalsis—coordinated waves that help push stool toward the rectum for eventual elimination.

When constipation occurs, several disruptions may take place during this process. A frequently cited cause is a slowing of intestinal transit, which happens when the colon's contractions are not as effective as they should be. This can result from a variety of factors, including a diet low in fiber–an essential nutrient that adds bulk to stool–and insufficient physical activity, which plays a critical role in stimulating healthy bowel movement. Other contributors may include stress and specific medications, both of which can adversely impact bowel function and slow digestion.

Constipation can also occur if the colon absorbs too much water from food waste. When the colon extracts more water than necessary, the resulting stool becomes dry and hard, making it difficult to pass. This is often linked to poor hydration. If we do not drink enough water or lose significant fluids through sweat, urination, or other means, the body responds by conserving water, which leads to hardened stool and more challenging elimination.

Furthermore, some medical conditions may exacerbate constipation. Neurological disorders, such as Parkinson's disease or multiple sclerosis, can interfere with the communication between the brain and the intestinal muscles responsible for colon contractions. Hormonal imbalances, including hypothyroidism, can also slow metabolism, which is closely associated with digestive efficiency.

Constipation can affect individuals across all ages, from children to adults, and its impact reaches far beyond the frequency of bowel movements. Common symptoms include excessive straining during defecation, dry and hard stools that cause discomfort or even pain, a sensation of incomplete bowel evacuation, abdominal bloating, and an overall feeling of heaviness. These symptoms not only lead to physical discomfort but can also take a toll on emotional well-being and self-esteem. Therefore, it is critical to recognize that this problem is solvable and should never be accepted as an unavoidable condition.

An often-overlooked but equally significant factor in chronic constipation lies in pelvic floor health. This group of muscles and tissues supports essential organs such as the rectum and anus and plays an integral role in stool elimination. Weakness, injury, or tension in the pelvic floor muscles can hinder their ability to function properly during defecation. This issue can worsen constipation and often requires specialized attention to manage effectively.

Despite its challenges, the encouraging news is that constipation can be managed and even overcome with a variety of effective strategies. This book serves as a complete and empowering guide to understanding this common health issue. Inside, you'll find clear and practical medical information, including definitions, types, potential causes, symptoms, and important warning signs to watch out for. Moreover, it offers actionable advice, diagnostic options, and complementary solutions–spanning a nutritious diet, targeted nutritional supplements, and medicinal plants–all designed to enhance your daily well-being. More than just a source of information, this book is your companion on the path towards a healthier, more comfortable life. If you've struggled with frustration or discomfort due to this condition, let this be your invitation to take control of your health. Small, practical changes can lead to meaningful results. Your journey to improved intestinal wellness begins here, and this book is ready to support you every step of the way.

## Types of Constipation

Constipation is a digestive condition that can manifest in different ways, depending on its causes and specific characteristics. Gaining a clear understanding of these variations is crucial for identifying the potential underlying factors and determining the most effective treatment. Below is an overview of the most common types of constipation:

▸ **Occasional constipation**: This is the most common type of constipation, characterized by sporadic episodes of difficulty passing stool. It may be related to changes in diet, lack of physical activity, travel, stress, or insufficient fluid intake. This type of constipation typically resolves on its own with temporary lifestyle and dietary adjustments.

▸ **Chronic constipation**: It is defined as the presence of constipation symptoms for at least three months. It may result from factors such as a low-fiber diet, lack of regular physical activity, insufficient fluid intake, medications, digestive system disorders, hormonal imbalances, or structural problems in the colon. This type of constipation often requires long-term changes in lifestyle and diet, as well as medical intervention to address the underlying causes.

▸ **Slow-transit constipation**: In this type of constipation, the stool moves slowly through the digestive tract. This may be due to various factors, including a low-fiber diet, a lack of physical activity, hormonal imbalances, or underlying medical conditions. Stools tend to be hard and dry, and bowel movements may require excessive straining. Treatment may include dietary changes, increased physical activity, and, in some cases, medications that stimulate bowel movements.

▸ **Obstructive constipation**: This type of constipation occurs when a physical obstruction in the bowel prevents the typical passage of stool. It may be the result of fecal impaction, a tumor, intestinal stricture, or a hernia. Obstructive constipation is a severe condition that requires immediate medical attention. Treatment may involve removing the obstruction through medical or surgical procedures.

▸ **Secondary constipation**: This type occurs due to an underlying medical condition. It may be associated with digestive system disorders, such as irritable bowel syndrome, inflammatory bowel disease, Parkinson's disease, or hypothyroidism. Treatment of secondary constipation focuses on addressing the underlying cause and may require specific medications, hormone therapy, or other medical approaches.

▸ **Constipation during pregnancy**: Many women experience constipation during pregnancy due to hormonal changes, increased pressure in the abdomen, and the growing uterus. In addition, the use of prenatal iron supplements can contribute to constipation. To alleviate this type of constipation, it is recommended to increase fiber intake, drink enough water, and exercise regularly, always under the supervision of a health care professional.

▸ **Constipation in children**: Children may also experience constipation, particularly during the transition to solid foods or during the potty training process. This may be due to a low-fiber diet, inadequate hydration, fecal impaction, or emotional factors such as stress or anxiety. In these cases, it is essential to encourage a balanced, high-fiber diet, ensure adequate hydration, and establish regular toileting routines.

▸ **Idiopathic constipation**: In some cases, constipation has no clear identifiable cause and is known as idiopathic or functional constipation. It may result from a combination of factors, such as a low-fiber diet, lack of physical activity, changes in lifestyle habits, nervous system disorders, or bowel muscle dysfunction. Treatment of idiopathic constipation usually involves dietary and lifestyle changes, along with medications and therapies specific to individual needs.

▸ **Medicated constipation**: Some medications can cause constipation as a side effect. These include opioids, analgesics, antidepressants, antipsychotics, antihypertensives, antacids with calcium or aluminum, and some iron supplements. Suppose you suspect that a medication is causing constipation. In that case, it is essential to consult your doctor to evaluate the possibility of adjusting the dose, changing the medication, or exploring alternatives.

## Symptoms

The symptoms of constipation can differ based on the specific type and severity of the condition. Recognizing these signs is key to accurately identifying the problem and adopting an effective management approach. The most common symptoms associated with various types of constipation are outlined below:

▸ **Occasional constipation**: This type of constipation is usually characterized by isolated episodes of difficulty passing stool. Symptoms may include excessive straining during bowel movements, hard and dry stools, a feeling of incomplete evacuation, and the need for extra effort to pass stool. In addition, abdominal discomfort, bloating, gas and fullness may be experienced after meals.

▸ **Chronic constipation**: Chronic constipation is the presence of symptoms for at least three months. In addition to the symptoms mentioned above, chronic constipation may cause other symptoms, such as abdominal pain, a feeling of blockage or difficulty passing stool, the need to use laxatives regularly, changes in stool consistency, and decreased frequency of bowel movements.

▸ **Slow transit constipation**: In this type of constipation, the stool moves slowly through the bowel. Symptoms may include infrequent bowel movements (less than three times per week), hard and dry stools, excessive straining during bowel movements, a feeling of incomplete evacuation, and abdominal distention. In addition, there may be a feeling of blockage in the rectum and the need to use enemas or suppositories to achieve evacuation.

▸ **Obstructive constipation**: Obstructive constipation is characterized by a physical obstruction in the bowel that prevents the normal passage of stool. Symptoms may include severe abdominal pain, abdominal bloating, nausea and vomiting, lack of appetite, unexplained weight loss, and the inability to pass stool or gas. This type of constipation is a medical emergency and requires immediate medical attention.

▸ **Secondary constipation**: Secondary constipation occurs when an underlying medical condition causes it. Symptoms may vary depending on the cause, but they may include hard, dry stools, straining during bowel movements, bloating, changes in the consistency and frequency of bowel movements, and other symptoms associated with the condition, such as abdominal pain in irritable bowel syndrome or diarrhea in inflammatory bowel disease.

▸ **Constipation in pregnancy**: In addition to the general symptoms of constipation, pregnant women may experience other related symptoms. These may include hemorrhoids due to the additional pressure on the anal region, as well as bloating and abdominal cramping. Some women may also experience pain during bowel movements due to pressure on the uterus.

▸ **Constipation in children**: The symptoms of constipation in children can vary depending on their age. Infants may present with crying and discomfort when trying to defecate, hard and dry stools, a lack of appetite, and difficulty sleeping. In older children, symptoms may include abdominal pain, fecal impaction, large and painful stools, and behavioral changes, such as avoiding using the toilet or hiding to defecate.

▸ **Idiopathic constipation**: In the case of idiopathic constipation, symptoms may be similar to those of chronic constipation. However, the duration and frequency of symptoms may vary. Some people may experience mild, occasional symptoms, while others may have persistent, severe symptoms. Additional symptoms related to the digestive system, such as heartburn, gas and general discomfort, may also occur.

▸ **Drug constipation**: The symptoms of drug constipation may be similar to occasional or chronic constipation. However, it is essential to note that symptoms may vary depending on the specific medication used. Some medicines may cause more severe constipation or be associated with other symptoms, such as changes in appetite or additional side effects. It is always advisable to consult a physician if a medication is suspected of causing constipation.

Each person may experience constipation differently. Symptoms can also vary in intensity or be accompanied by additional signs depending on the situation. If there are any concerns about the symptoms, or if constipation becomes persistent, it is essential to seek medical attention for an accurate diagnosis.

# Causes

Constipation can result from a variety of causes, ranging from temporary factors to chronic conditions. Gaining a clear understanding of these causes is essential for identifying the root of the issue and addressing it effectively. Below are the primary causes of constipation:

- **Low fiber diet**: One of the leading causes of constipation is a diet low in fiber. Fiber helps keep stool soft and bulky, making it easier to pass through the intestine. Insufficient intake of fruits, vegetables, whole grains and legumes can contribute to constipation.

- **Insufficient fluid intake**: Dehydration and inadequate fluid intake can cause stools to become complex and difficult to pass. Drinking enough water and other fluids is crucial for maintaining adequate hydration and promoting regular bowel movements.

- **Lack of physical activity**: Sedentary lifestyles and a lack of physical activity can affect intestinal motility and contribute to constipation. Regular exercise helps stimulate the movement of intestinal muscles, facilitating the passage of stool through the intestine.

- **Lifestyle factors**: Lifestyle factors, such as a lack of time to use the bathroom, suppression of the urge to defecate, stress, and changes in daily routine, can contribute to constipation. These factors can disrupt standard bowel movement patterns, making it challenging to pass stool regularly.

- **Medications**: Some medications can cause constipation as a side effect. These can include opioids, antacids containing calcium or aluminum, some blood pressure medications, antidepressants, and medications to treat certain neurological conditions. If you suspect that a medication is causing constipation, it is essential to talk to your doctor to evaluate alternatives or adjust the dosage.

- **Structural problems or blockages**: Constipation can also be caused by structural problems in the bowel that make it difficult for stool to pass. This may include intestinal obstructions, intestinal strictures (narrowing), hernias, or tumors. These conditions require immediate medical attention.

▸ **Diseases and disorders**: Several diseases and disorders may be associated with constipation. Examples include irritable bowel syndrome, inflammatory bowel disease (such as Crohn's disease and ulcerative colitis), diabetes, hypothyroidism, multiple sclerosis, and neuromuscular disorders.

▸ **Hormonal changes**: In some women, hormonal changes during the menstrual cycle, pregnancy, or menopause may influence bowel regularity and cause temporary constipation.

▸ **Psychological factors**: Stress, anxiety and depression can affect the normal functioning of the digestive system and contribute to constipation.

▸ **Changes in lifestyle habits**: Daily routines, such as traveling or adapting to new work schedules, can disrupt regular bowel movement patterns and contribute to constipation. The body often requires time to adjust to these changes and restore a normal rhythm.

▸ **Muscle and nerve disorders**: Problems affecting the muscles and nerves in the bowel can interfere with bowel motility, leading to constipation. These issues may arise from conditions such as irritable bowel syndrome, neurological disorders, spinal cord injuries, or nerve damage that impacts bowel control.

▸ **Metabolic disorders**: Some metabolic disorders, such as hypothyroidism and diabetes, can affect bowel function and cause constipation. These conditions can alter hormonal balance and affect intestinal motility.

▸ **Anatomical structural problems**: Some people may have structural abnormalities in the bowel that make it difficult for them to pass stool. This may include narrowing (strictures), obstructions or blockages in the bowel, polyps, or intestinal diverticula. These conditions may require medical or surgical intervention to correct the problem.

▸ **Pelvic floor disorders**: The pelvic floor is a group of muscles that help control bowel movements and urination. Pelvic floor disorders, such as pelvic floor dysfunction or muscle weakness, can interfere with normal bowel function and cause constipation.

▸ **Aging**: As we age, bowel function often becomes less efficient, which can contribute to constipation. Decreased physical activity, dietary changes, and age-related medical conditions may be contributing factors.

▸ **Emotional and psychological factors**: Stress, anxiety and depression can affect bowel function and contribute to constipation. The nervous and digestive systems are interconnected, and emotions can influence intestinal motility.

It is important to remember that each person may have different causes of constipation, and multiple factors are often involved.

## Potential Complications

*This section is designed to offer clear guidance and effectively highlight potential risks, with an emphasis on prevention. By doing so, you can take proactive steps to safeguard your well-being and minimize the likelihood of complications.*

Chronic constipation, if not properly managed, can result in various complications that may significantly affect your quality of life. Below are some of the most common health issues associated with persistent constipation:

▸ **Hemorrhoids**: Excessive straining during bowel movements due to constipation can cause hemorrhoids. Hemorrhoids are swollen veins in the rectum and anus that can cause pain, itching and bleeding. Repetitive straining during bowel movements increases pressure in the rectal veins, which can lead to the development or worsening of hemorrhoids.

▸ **Anal fissures**: Anal fissures are small breaks or tears in the skin of the anal canal. Chronic constipation can cause anal fissures to form due to the passage of hard, bulky stool through the anal canal. This can cause severe pain during bowel movements and rectal bleeding.

▸ **Fecal impaction**: Fecal impaction occurs when stool accumulates and hardens in the rectum, making it difficult to pass. It can occur in people with severe chronic constipation and can cause abdominal pain, bloating, loss of appetite, and bowel obstruction.

▸ **Diverticulosis**: Diverticulosis is when small pouches or sacs form in the colon's wall. Chronic constipation can increase colon pressure, contributing to the development of diverticula. If the diverticula become inflamed or infected, a condition known as diverticulitis occurs, which can cause severe abdominal pain, fever and other symptoms.

▸ **Megacolon**: Chronic, untreated constipation can cause an abnormal enlargement of the colon, known as megacolon. In megacolon, the colon becomes enlarged and weakened, making it difficult for the stool to pass. This can lead to increased stool retention and an increased risk of complications, such as bowel obstruction.

▸ **Fecal incontinence**: In some cases, chronic constipation can lead to fecal incontinence, which is the inability to control the passage of stool. The accumulation of hardened stool in the rectum can put pressure on the anal muscles, weakening them and leading to involuntary leakage of liquid or solid stool.

▸ **Development of polyps and colon cancer**: If constipation persists for a long time, it can increase the risk of developing colorectal polyps and abnormal growths in the colon's lining. If polyps are not detected and removed in time, they can develop into colon cancer.

▸ **Urinary problems**: Chronic constipation can pressure the bladder and nearby organs, affecting urinary function. This can cause difficulty urinating, recurrent urinary tract infections, or loss of bladder control.

▸ **Irritable bowel syndrome (IBS)**: Chronic constipation can be a symptom of IBS, a chronic digestive system condition characterized by abdominal pain, bloating, changes in bowel habits, and general discomfort. Constipation in IBS can be debilitating and significantly affect a person's quality of life.

▸ **Impact on quality of life**: Chronic constipation can significantly impact a person's quality of life. Physical discomfort, abdominal pain, bloating, and a feeling of fullness can make daily activities difficult. In addition, constipation can cause anxiety, stress and frustration, which can affect a person's mental and emotional health.

▸ **Nutrient absorption problems**: When stool remains in the intestine for prolonged periods due to constipation, the proper absorption of nutrients can decrease. This can lead to nutritional deficiencies and several health problems, including weakness, fatigue, weight loss, and malnutrition.

▸ **Increased risk of cardiovascular disease**: Some studies have suggested an association between chronic constipation and an increased risk of cardiovascular diseases, such as heart disease, stroke and high blood pressure. While the exact relationship is not fully understood, it is believed that chronic inflammation and gut microbiota imbalances may contribute to this connection.

▸ **Impact on mental health**: Chronic constipation can have a significant effect on a person's mental and emotional health. Physical discomfort, discomfort and constant worry can contribute to stress, anxiety and depression. In addition, the feeling of not having a proper bowel movement can lead to frustration, irritability and low self-esteem.

▸ **Complications during pregnancy**: Constipation is common due to hormonal changes, increased pressure on the bowel due to the growing uterus, and absorption of extra fluids. However, chronic and untreated constipation may increase the risk of hemorrhoids, anal fissures and general discomfort during pregnancy.

## Symptom Relief and Prevention

Addressing symptoms and preventing constipation are vital for maintaining optimal digestive health. Implementing targeted strategies and making lifestyle adjustments can make a significant difference. Here are key recommendations to consider:

▸ **Adequate fiber intake**: Fiber is crucial for maintaining a healthy digestive system and preventing constipation. Adults should aim to consume at least 25-30 grams of fiber daily. Excellent sources of fiber include fruits, vegetables, legumes, whole grains, and nuts. Gradually increasing fiber intake allows the body to adjust, helping to regulate bowel movements and soften stool, making it easier to pass through the digestive tract.

▸ **Stay Hydrated**: Dehydration can worsen constipation, as water plays a key role in softening stool and facilitating its smooth passage through the intestines. It is generally recommended to drink at least 8 glasses of water daily; however, individual hydration needs may vary depending on factors such as age, weight, physical activity, and climate. Staying properly hydrated is essential for healthy bowel function.

▸ **Maintain an active lifestyle**: Regular physical activity can help stimulate bowel movements and prevent constipation. Activities such as walking, running, swimming, or yoga can promote bowel motility and improve the regularity of bowel movements. Try to get at least 30 minutes of moderate exercise most days of the week.

▸ **Establish a regular bowel routine**: Set aside sufficient time to use the bathroom regularly. The body tends to follow patterns, so going to the bathroom at the same time every day can help regularize bowel movements.

▸ **Avoid a sedentary lifestyle**: Sitting for long periods or being inactive can slow down bowel transit and contribute to constipation. Try to move around and get up regularly throughout the day, especially if you have a job that requires you to sit for long periods. Simple stretches or short walks help stimulate the bowel and prevent stool stagnation.

▸ **Avoid excessive use of laxatives**: While laxatives can be helpful in cases of occasional constipation, excessive or prolonged use can cause dependence and damage natural bowel function. It is essential to consult a physician before taking any laxatives and use them only as directed.

▸ **Manage stress**: Chronic stress can affect bowel function and contribute to constipation. Finding ways to manage stress, such as practicing relaxation techniques, meditation, yoga, or seeking professional psychological support, can have a positive impact on digestive health.

▸ **Avoid medication abuse**: Some medications, such as opioid pain relievers, antidepressants, and antacids containing calcium or aluminum, can contribute to constipation. If you are taking medicines that may be related to constipation, talk to your doctor about possible alternatives or strategies to minimize this side effect.

▸ **Balanced diet**: In addition to increasing fiber intake, it is essential to maintain a balanced diet that includes a variety of healthy foods. Eating fresh fruits and vegetables, whole grains, lean proteins and healthy fats can help maintain proper bowel function. Avoid processed foods high in saturated fats and added sugars, which can contribute to constipation.

▸ **Probiotics**: Probiotics are beneficial microorganisms that help maintain a healthy balance in the gut microbiota, which is essential for proper digestion and gut function. You can find probiotics in foods such as yogurt, kefir and sauerkraut, or you may also choose to take probiotic supplements. Consult with a healthcare professional to determine what type and dosage of probiotics may be right for you.

▸ **Avoid excessive alcohol and caffeine consumption**: Both alcohol and caffeine can contribute to constipation. Alcohol can dehydrate you and affect intestinal motility, while caffeine can act as a diuretic, increasing fluid excretion and potentially triggering constipation. Limit your consumption of these substances and stay hydrated if you choose to consume them.

▸ **Please do not ignore the urge to evacuate**: It is essential to listen to your body's signals and not ignore the urge to evacuate when needed. Withholding stool can lead to hardening and accumulation, making it difficult to pass later. If you feel the urge to go to the bathroom, find a nearby restroom and take the time necessary for a complete bowel movement.

▸ **Avoid excessive use of enemas or suppositories**: Although they may be helpful in some cases of severe constipation, they should not be used habitually or excessively. Overuse of these methods can damage natural bowel function and cause dependency. Please consult a physician before using the medication and follow their recommendations.

▸ **Manage underlying health conditions**: Some health conditions, such as hypothyroidism, diabetes and colon disorders, can contribute to constipation. If you have any underlying health conditions, it is essential to monitor them correctly and follow your doctor's recommendations to prevent and manage constipation effectively.

It is important to remember that every person is unique and may require personalized strategies to effectively prevent and manage constipation. If constipation persists, becomes severe, or does not improve despite lifestyle changes, do not hesitate to consult a healthcare professional for an accurate diagnosis and appropriate treatment.

## Additional Recommendations

In addition to the changes mentioned earlier, the following measures can help relieve and prevent constipation:

▸ **Try foods with laxative properties**: Certain foods contain natural laxative properties that can help relieve constipation. Examples include prunes, kiwi fruit, pears, figs, unsalted peanuts, olive oil, yogurt with probiotics, and apple juice with no added sugar. Including these foods in your diet can help stimulate bowel movements.

▸ **Avoid excessive consumption of foods that can cause constipation**: Some foods can worsen constipation, so it is advisable to limit their consumption. These include processed and refined foods, foods high in saturated fats, red meats, full-fat dairy products and low-fiber foods. Additionally, limit your intake of foods that may cause constipation in some people, such as green bananas or starchy foods.

▸ **Consider castor oil**: Castor oil is a natural laxative that can help soften stools and stimulate bowel movements. However, it is essential to use it with caution and under the supervision of a health professional, as it can have side effects and should not be used long-term.

▸ **Try abdominal relaxation techniques**: Gentle abdominal massage or applying heat to the abdominal area can help stimulate bowel movements and relieve constipation. Consult a health professional for proper instructions on how to perform these techniques.

▸ **To improve evacuation**, you can squat or sit on the toilet with your knees close to your chest, using a low stool to support your feet. Toilet stools are available for this purpose.

▸ **Laughing** is beneficial as it creates an abdominal massage effect that aids digestion.

▸ Additionally, **engaging in exercises that stimulate intestinal activity** is highly recommended. Below are two exercises that may help:

  - Lie on your back with your legs together and bent, resting your feet on the floor. Place your arms at your sides. Slowly raise your legs as far as possible, bringing your knees close to your abdomen. Hold this position for a few seconds and then slowly lower your legs without taking your back off the floor, returning to the starting position. Repeat this exercise 6 times.

- Lie on your back with your back on the floor and your legs bent at right angles. Place your hands on your knees. Keeping your legs together and without lifting your back off the floor, gently draw four circles in the air with the tips of your toes. Then, repeat the exercise in the opposite direction.

## Considerations Regarding Laxatives

Frequent or prolonged use of laxatives can pose significant health risks. While they may be effective for occasional episodes of constipation, overuse or dependence on these products can have harmful consequences. Below are some of the primary contraindications and side effects:

▸ **Dependence and tolerance**: Frequent use of laxatives can lead to dependence, where the body becomes accustomed to the laxative and requires increasing amounts to achieve the same effect. This can cause the bowel to become sluggish and dependent on laxatives to function correctly. Dependence on laxatives can hinder the natural process of evacuation and worsen constipation in the long run.

▸ **Damage to the digestive system**: Prolonged use of laxatives can damage the digestive system. Stimulant laxatives, in particular, can irritate the intestinal mucosa and cause inflammation. This can lead to problems such as colitis, inflammatory bowel disease, or colon dysfunction. In addition, laxatives can interfere with the absorption of essential nutrients, such as fat-soluble vitamins, minerals and electrolytes, leading to nutritional deficiencies.

▸ **Dehydration**: Some laxatives, such as osmotic laxatives and stimulant laxatives, can cause dehydration due to their mechanism of action. These laxatives draw water into the bowel to soften the stool, which can result in excessive fluid loss in the body. Dehydration can have a negative impact on overall health and exacerbate constipation in the long term.

▸ **Electrolyte imbalance**: Prolonged use of laxatives can also upset the balance of electrolytes, such as potassium, sodium and magnesium. Electrolytes are essential for the proper functioning of the nervous system, muscles, and other organs. Electrolyte imbalance can cause muscle weakness, cramps, heart arrhythmias and other health problems.

▸ **Damage to the intestinal flora**: Excessive use of laxatives can negatively impact the intestinal flora, a community of beneficial bacteria that inhabit the intestine and play a crucial role in maintaining digestive health. Laxatives can disrupt the balance of intestinal bacteria, negatively affecting digestion, nutrient absorption and immune function.

▸ **Rebound effect**: A rebound effect can occur when laxative use is discontinued after prolonged use. This means that the bowel may become even more sluggish, and constipation may temporarily worsen due to the dependence that develops from the use of laxatives.

▸ **Loss of muscle tone and function**: Prolonged use of laxatives can weaken the bowel muscles, reducing normal peristaltic movement function. This can cause the bowel to become less efficient in moving stool through the digestive tract, worsening long-term constipation.

▸ **Alterations in medication absorption**: Some laxatives can interfere with the absorption of oral medications. This is because laxatives can speed up the passage of food and substances through the intestine, which does not allow enough time for drugs to be absorbed properly. This can reduce the effectiveness of certain medications and compromise their treatment.

▸ **Increased risk of nutritional imbalances**: The continued or frequent use of laxatives can interfere with the absorption of essential vitamins and minerals, thereby increasing the risk of nutritional imbalances. Nutritional deficiencies can occur if these essential nutrients are not adequately supplemented through a balanced diet. Nutrient deficiencies can negatively affect overall health and worsen constipation-related symptoms.

▸ **Alterations in kidney function**: Some laxatives, especially those containing magnesium salts or sodium phosphate, can increase the kidney load and affect their normal function. They can also cause dehydration and electrolyte imbalances, which can put additional stress on the kidneys and increase the risk of kidney damage.

▸ **Drug interactions**: Some laxatives may interact with other medications you are taking, decreasing their effectiveness or increasing the risk of side effects. It is essential to inform your doctor or pharmacist of all medications you are taking, including laxatives, to avoid possible harmful interactions.

▸ **Worsening of underlying health conditions**: Continued or frequent use of laxatives may worsen underlying health conditions, such as inflammatory bowel disease, irritable bowel syndrome, or Crohn's disease. These conditions can already cause digestive disorders, and inappropriate laxative use can aggravate symptoms and complicate the management of these diseases.

It is important to emphasize that these contraindications primarily pertain to the prolonged or excessive use of laxatives, not their occasional and controlled use under the guidance of a healthcare professional. If you experience chronic constipation, it is vital to consult your doctor to identify and address the under-lying cause. Adopting a comprehensive and safe approach is far more effective than relying solely on laxatives as a solution.

## Diagnostic Medical Tests

Healthcare professionals have a variety of tests at their disposal to investigate the underlying causes of constipation. These evaluations are essential for establishing an accurate diagnosis and determining the most appropriate treatment.

Below is an overview of the most commonly used tests:

▸ **Medical history and physical examination**: Your doctor will begin by taking a detailed medical history and asking you questions about your symptoms, including their duration, frequency, and severity. They may also ask about your medical history, medications, eating habits and general lifestyle. The doctor will then perform a physical examination to assess your abdomen, check for masses or tenderness, and identify signs of bowel obstruction or distension.

▸ **Blood tests**: Blood tests may be ordered to evaluate thyroid function, as impaired thyroid function may contribute to constipation. Blood electrolyte levels, such as potassium and calcium, may also be measured, as electrolyte imbalances may be related to constipation.

▸ **Imaging tests**: Imaging tests can help identify structural problems in the digestive system that may be causing constipation. The most common tests include:

- *Simple abdominal X-ray*: It is used to evaluate the presence of obstructions, colon enlargement, or fecal impaction.

- *Barium enema*: Used to evaluate the rectum and colon by administering a contrast liquid (barium) that allows the bowel lining to be visualized on an X-ray.

- *Colonoscopy*: This procedure uses a flexible camera to visually inspect the lining of the colon and rectum. It can detect polyps, tumors, inflammation, or other abnormalities that may cause constipation.

▸ **Anorectal manometry**: This test measures the activity and function of the anal sphincter and rectal muscles. It is used to assess muscle tone and the ability of the muscles to coordinate proper evacuation of stool.

▸ **Colonic transit**: This test evaluates the time it takes for food to pass through the large intestine. You will be asked to swallow capsules containing radiopaque tracers, and then X-rays will be taken at timed intervals to track the movement of the tracers through the intestine.

▸ **Air balloon expulsion test**: This test assesses the rectum's ability to expel an inflated balloon. A small balloon is inserted into the rectum, and you are asked to expel it. This helps determine if rectal dysfunction is contributing to constipation.

▸ **Gastrointestinal transit test**: This test evaluates the time it takes for food to move through the entire gastrointestinal tract. You will be asked to swallow a capsule or a food marked with a radiopaque material, and then x-rays will be taken at timed intervals to track the movement of markers throughout the digestive system. This test helps identify if there is a delay in bowel transit, which can contribute to constipation.

▸ **Esophageal manometry**: This test evaluates the function of the esophagus to determine if any motility problems may affect the passage of food from the esophagus to the stomach. Although it is not a specific test for constipation, it can rule out problems in the esophagus that may contribute to chronic constipation.

▸ **Hydrogen breath test**: This test assesses the presence of lactose intolerance or food allergies, which can cause symptoms of constipation. You will be asked to drink a solution containing lactose or a specific food, and then the amount of hydrogen in your breath will be measured. An increase in hydrogen levels may indicate a food intolerance or allergy.

▸ **Colonic motility study**: This test evaluates the function and coordination of the colon muscles. A flexible tube is inserted through the rectum, and the contractions and movements of the colon are measured. This helps identify possible motility issues that may be contributing to constipation.

▸ **Defecography test**: This test is used to evaluate the function of the rectum and anus during the defecation process. X-ray or MRI images are obtained while you are asked to strain to defecate. This allows the rectum, anus, and surrounding muscles to be evaluated for any structural or functional problems that may contribute to constipation.

It is essential to understand that not all of these tests are required in every case of constipation. Your doctor will evaluate your symptoms, medical history, and physical examination to determine which tests are most appropriate for your specific situation. In some instances, a combination of tests may be necessary to arrive at an accurate diagnosis.

## Warning Signs

Occasional constipation is common and, in most cases, is not a serious concern. However, certain symptoms may indicate more severe conditions that require immediate medical attention. The key warning signs to watch for are outlined below:

▸ **Presence of Blood in Stool**: The appearance of dried blood or dark clots in stool may indicate internal bleeding in the upper digestive tract.
Bright red blood, on the other hand, may suggest hemorrhoids or anal fissures. However, it could also be a sign of more serious conditions, such as polyps, colitis, or even colorectal cancer in severe cases.

▸ **Unexplained Weight Loss**: A significant, unexplained reduction in weight–without any changes to diet or physical activity–could be a warning sign of an underlying health issue, such as a metabolic disorder, chronic infections, or cancer.

▸ **Anemia**: Anemia, particularly when accompanied by constipation, may stem from hidden bleeding in the gastrointestinal tract. Possible causes include conditions like gastrointestinal ulcers or tumors.

▸ **Relevant Family History**: Having close relatives diagnosed with conditions such as colon cancer or inflammatory bowel diseases (e.g., Crohn's disease or ulcerative colitis) increases your risk of developing serious complications. This under-scores the importance of early and comprehensive medical evaluation.

▸ **Severe Abdominal Distension**: Marked abdominal bloating or distension could be indicative of an intestinal obstruction, a condition that blocks the normal passage of intestinal contents. Prompt medical intervention is essential to avoid severe complications.

▸ **Sudden Onset of Symptoms in Individuals Over 50**: The sudden and persistent onset of severe constipation in people over 50 warrants immediate investigation. This could be associated with serious conditions such as colorectal cancer, diverticulitis, or other age-related gastrointestinal issues.

▸ **Other Warning Symptoms:**
  - Persistent or severe abdominal pain.
  - High fever, which may signify an infection or inflamma-tion.
  - Significant, long-lasting changes in bowel habits, such as alternating between constipation and diarrhea.

**What to Do If You Notice These Signs:**
If you experience any of these warning signs, it is vital to consult your doctor as soon as possible. Early detection and treatment can significantly influence the outcome of potentially serious medical conditions. Be sure to provide your healthcare provider with a detailed account of your symptoms and medical history to facilitate an accurate diagnosis.

## Symptoms of appendicitis

Appendicitis is a painful and infectious inflammation of the appendix, a small, tube-shaped organ attached to the large intestine. This is a medical condition that can quickly become severe if not treated promptly. Although symptoms may vary among individuals, the primary signs of appendicitis include:

▸ **Abdominal pain:**
  - Onset of pain: Discomfort typically begins in the central

abdominal area, near or around the belly button.
- Migration of pain: Over time, the pain shifts to the lower right side of the abdomen, particularly near an area known as McBurney's point.
- Nature of the pain: The pain is usually constant, progressive, and intense. It tends to worsen with movement, coughing, sneezing, or even walking.

▸ **Abdominal tenderness**:
- Pressing or touching the area over the appendix often causes sharp pain or localized tenderness.
- Rebound tenderness: Some individuals experience increased pain when pressure is quickly released from the abdomen.Pressure or touch in the area of the appendix may cause tenderness or sharp pain.

▸ **Loss of appetite**: Inflammation of the appendix often leads to a noticeable loss of appetite, mainly due to abdominal discomfort and intestinal dysfunction.

▸ **Nausea and vomiting**: People with appendicitis frequently experience nausea accompanied by vomiting. These symptoms usually occur shortly after the abdominal pain begins.

▸ **Fever**:
- Appendicitis can cause a mild fever, typically ranging between 99.5°F and 100.4°F (37.5°C-38°C), often accompanied by chills.
- A higher fever may indicate complications, such as a ruptured appendix or a more severe infection.

▸ **Changes in bowel habits**:
- Alterations in bowel movements, such as constipation or mild diarrhea, may occur.
- Some individuals may struggle to pass gas, which can lead to bloating and increased discomfort.

**Key Factors to Consider**
The symptoms and severity of appendicitis can vary signi-

ficantly depending on factors such as age, individual health, and the stage of the condition.

- Young children and older adults: Symptoms may be less pronounced in these groups, making diagnosis more difficult.
- Pregnancy: Pregnant women may experience pain in a slightly different location because the growing uterus displaces the appendix.

### Why Is It Urgent to Treat Appendicitis?

Appendicitis is a medical emergency that can become life-threatening if left untreated. Without prompt intervention, the inflamed appendix may:

- Rupture (burst appendix): This allows infectious material to spill into the abdominal cavity, leading to peritonitis–a severe, widespread infection.
- Form abscesses: Pockets of pus may develop around the appendix, increasing the risk of complications.

### Key Recommendation

If you experience symptoms consistent with appendicitis, do not wait for them to subside on their own, as the condition can worsen rapidly. Seek urgent medical attention for an accurate diagnosis and, if necessary, timely surgical intervention to address the problem effectively.

# FREQUENTLY ASKED QUESTIONS

Navigating the intricate world of health can be a challenging experience, especially when faced with a diagnosis that impacts both your body and emotions. In such moments, many questions arise: What are the implications? What options are available? How will my daily life change? These and other concerns are common in situations like this. Here, you'll find practical and straightforward answers to help you make informed decisions with greater confidence.

This chapter is born out of a desire to provide support and clear tools to help you navigate this path with confidence. In an era overflowing with information–though not always reliable–it's crucial to distinguish between valuable insights and those that may create confusion. For this reason, I have compiled evidence-based answers to guide you through moments of uncertainty.

The question-and-answer format has been thoughtfully designed with practicality in mind, addressing the most common concerns faced by individuals and their families. The explanations are simple, concise, and focused on facilitating decisions that prioritize your well-being.

While the information presented here aims to be helpful, it is not a substitute for personalized medical advice. It's always essential to consult with your doctor to address specific issues that may arise.

Through these pages, I hope to offer tranquility, confidence, and steadfast support to help you face challenges with resilience. My goal is for this resource to inspire you and equip you with the tools needed to confidently confront this condition.

# 109 FAQs about Constipation

### 1. What is constipation?

Constipation is characterized by fewer than three bowel movements per week or those that are difficult or painful to pass. It may include hard, dry stools and is often accompanied by a feeling of incomplete evacuation.

### 2. What are the common causes of constipation?

A low-fiber diet can cause constipation, lack of physical activity, dehydration, certain medications, changes in daily routine, or underlying diseases such as irritable bowel syndrome, among others.

### 3. When should I see my doctor for constipation?

A physician should be consulted if constipation is persistent, if there is severe pain, blood in the stool, unexplained weight loss, or if there are significant changes in bowel habits.

### 4. How can constipation be prevented?

To prevent constipation, eat a diet rich in fiber, drink plenty of water, engage in regular physical activity, and establish a regular bathroom routine, among other measures.

### 5. How can stress affect constipation?

Stress can negatively influence the digestive system by altering intestinal motility, the secretion of hormones and neurotransmitters that regulate intestinal transit, and the perception of abdominal pain. Stress management techniques, such as meditation, cognitive behavioral therapy, deep breathing, and yoga, can help relieve stress-related constipation.

### 6. What are osmotic laxatives, and how do they work?

Osmotic laxatives, such as polyethylene glycol (PEG) and lactulose, work by retaining water in the intestine, which softens the stool and makes it easier to pass. They effectively relieve occasional constipation and are generally safe for short-term use.

### 7. What are bulk-forming laxatives, and how do they work?

Bulk-forming laxatives, such as psyllium, absorb water in the intestine. This increases stool bulk and stimulates intestinal transit. They are generally safe for long-term use, but consuming them with sufficient water is essential.

### 8. Is the prolonged use of laxatives recommended to treat constipation?

Prolonged use of laxatives can lead to physical dependence, where the bowel loses its ability to function normally without them, damage to the bowel, and electrolyte imbalances. It is vital to use them under medical supervision and only when necessary, or to seek natural alternatives and explore changes in diet and lifestyle.

### 9. What are the differences between acute and chronic constipation?

Acute constipation is a temporary condition typically related to changes in diet or lifestyle. Chronic constipation is persistent and may require a more comprehensive approach to identify and treat the underlying causes.

### 10. How is constipation diagnosed?

The diagnosis of constipation is typically based on a medical history and a physical examination. However, in some cases, additional tests, such as blood tests, proctography, defecography, or colonic transit tests, may be necessary.

### 11. What is proctography, and how is it used to diagnose constipation?

Proctography is an imaging test that evaluates the function of the rectum and anus during bowel movements. It is used to diagnose structural or functional problems contributing to constipation.

### 12. What is defecography, and how is it used to diagnose constipation?

Defecography is an imaging test that evaluates the function of the rectum and anus during defecation. It helps identify problems such as rectal prolapse or pelvic floor dysfunction that could be contributing to constipation.

### 13. What is the colonic transit test?

Colonic transit testing evaluates the time it takes for stool to move through the colon. It can be performed using radiopaque markers ingested and then observed through X-rays to help diagnose bowel motility problems that may be causing constipation.

### 14. What is sigmoidoscopy, and how is it used to diagnose constipation?

Sigmoidoscopy is a procedure in which a thin tube with a camera examines the inside of the sigmoid colon and rectum to identify structural or inflammatory problems that may be causing constipation.

### 15. How does dehydration affect constipation?

Dehydration can make passing stools more challenging as the body absorbs more water from the intestines. Drinking enough water daily is essential to maintaining proper bowel function.

### 16. What impact does caffeine consumption have on constipation?

Caffeine's natural laxative effect can help stimulate bowel movements in some people. However, it can also contribute to dehydration, so balancing consumption with sufficient water is essential.

### 17. Does alcohol consumption affect constipation?

Alcohol can dehydrate the body, which can lead to drier stools that are more difficult to pass, contributing to constipation. Consuming alcohol in moderation and increasing water intake may help.

### 18. How does pregnancy affect constipation?

Hormonal changes during pregnancy, such as a significant increase in progesterone, can slow intestinal transit. In addition, the intake of iron supplements and the pressure of the growing uterus on the bowel also often contribute to constipation.

### 19. Can constipation cause other health problems?

Chronic constipation can lead to complications such as hemorrhoids, anal fissures, and in severe cases, fecal impaction, among others. It can also affect quality of life due to abdominal discomfort and bloating.

### 20. What role do fiber supplements play in the management of constipation?

Fiber supplements, such as psyllium, can help increase the bulk and softness of the stool, making it easier to pass. They are a practical option for those who do not get enough fiber through their diet. However, it is important to gradually increase fiber intake and drink enough water.

### 21. How can soluble and insoluble fiber affect constipation?

Soluble fiber, found in foods such as oats, nuts and legumes, absorbs water and forms a gel that can help soften stool. Insoluble fiber in wheat bran and vegetables adds bulk to the stool and speeds its passage through the intestine. Both types are essential in preventing or improving constipation.

### 22. Can the use of probiotics improve constipation?

Probiotics can help balance intestinal flora and improve bowel regularity in some people. Choosing a probiotic supplement containing specific strains known for improving intestinal motility and stool consistency is advisable.

### 23. Can weight gain be related to constipation?

Weight gain may be related to constipation, which can occur when the body retains stool and fluid. However, constipation alone is not usually a direct cause of significant weight gain.

### 24. Does physical activity help with constipation?

Yes, regular physical activity helps stimulate the digestive system and can improve intestinal transit, which in turn helps prevent or alleviate constipation. You should incorporate exercises such as walking, running, swimming, or yoga into your daily routine to stay healthy.

### 25. How can lifestyle changes improve constipation?

Healthy habits, such as a fiber-rich diet, adequate hydration, regular exercise, and establishing a bathroom routine, can significantly improve constipation symptoms.

### 26. How do eating disorders influence constipation?

Eating disorders, such as anorexia nervosa and bulimia, can lead to insufficient nutrient intake, dehydration and electrolyte imbalances, which can cause or aggravate constipation. Treatment should address both the eating disorder and the digestive symptoms.

### 27. How can constipation in children be treated?

Treatment for constipation in children includes maintaining proper nutrition to prevent it, increasing fiber and water intake, encouraging regular exercise, and establishing a consistent bathroom routine. Under medical supervision, natural supplements or mild laxatives may be recommended occasionally.

### 28. Are there gender differences in the prevalence of constipation?

Constipation is more common in women than in men, possibly due to hormonal factors, differences in diet, and bowel structure.

### 29. Is constipation more common at any stage of life?

Constipation is common in all stages of life but is more frequent in the elderly, women (especially during pregnancy), and people with sedentary lifestyles.

### 30. How can hormonal changes affect constipation in women?

Hormonal changes, especially during the menstrual cycle, pregnancy, or menopause, can affect bowel transit and cause constipation in some women. Fluctuations in hormones such as estrogen and progesterone are contributing factors. Maintaining a proper healthy diet and lifestyle often helps mitigate these effects.

### 31. How does the menstrual cycle affect constipation?

Some women experience changes in bowel habits during the menstrual cycle due to hormonal fluctuations. This may include constipation before or during menstruation.

### 32. How does menopause affect constipation?

During menopause, hormonal changes can slow down bowel

transit and cause constipation. Staying active and eating a healthy, high-fiber diet can help manage these symptoms.

### 33. How does aging affect constipation?

With aging, intestinal motility may decrease, and older people may experience constipation more frequently due to reduced physical activity, dietary changes, and certain medications. Maintaining an adequate diet rich in fiber, drinking plenty of water, and engaging in regular physical activity (such as walking or swimming) can often help mitigate these effects.

### 34. Can the low-carbohydrate diet cause constipation?

Yes, a low-carbohydrate diet that lacks sufficient fiber can contribute to constipation. It is essential to incorporate sources of fiber, such as vegetables, seeds, and nuts, into any diet plan.

### 35. How does hypothyroidism affect constipation?

Hypothyroidism, a condition in which the thyroid gland does not produce enough hormones, can slow down bodily processes, including intestinal transit, leading to constipation.

### 36. How can food allergies contribute to constipation?

Food allergies or intolerances, such as gluten or lactose intolerance, can cause digestive problems, including constipation. Identifying and eliminating trigger foods from the diet can help alleviate symptoms.

### 37. Can gluten affect constipation?

In people with celiac disease or non-celiac gluten sensitivity, gluten consumption can cause symptoms such as constipation. Eliminating gluten from the diet may improve symptoms in these cases.

### 38. How does celiac disease affect constipation?

Celiac disease is an autoimmune reaction to gluten that damages the small intestine. Although often associated with diarrhea, some people with celiac disease experience constipation. Treatment involves following a strict gluten-free diet.

### 39. How can dairy consumption affect constipation?

For some people, especially those with lactose intolerance, excessive consumption of dairy products can contribute to constipation. Reducing dairy intake or opting for lactose-free alternatives may be beneficial.

### 40. What is the hydrogen breath test, and how is it used?
The hydrogen breath test measures the amount of hydrogen in the breath after consuming a specific sugar. It is used to diagnose food intolerances, such as lactose intolerance, which can cause gastrointestinal symptoms, including constipation.

### 41. What effect do some medications have on constipation?
Some medications, including opioid analgesics, antidepressants and iron supplements, can cause constipation as a side effect.

### 42. How can pain medications, such as opioids, contribute to constipation?
Opioids, used for pain management, can cause or worsen constipation by slowing bowel transit and increasing fluid absorption in the intestine, leading to more complex and more difficult-to-pass stools.

### 43. How do antidepressants influence constipation?
Some antidepressants, especially tricyclics, may cause constipation as a side effect by affecting the neurotransmitters that regulate intestinal motility. Adjusting the medication or switching to another type of antidepressant may be necessary.

### 44. What is the relationship between the use of iron supplements and constipation?
Iron supplements may cause constipation as a side effect, as iron can harden the stool. To minimize this effect, taking the supplement with food and staying well hydrated is recommended.

### 45. What role does the intestinal microbiota play in constipation?
The intestinal microbiota, composed of trillions of bacteria, influences digestion and intestinal motility. An imbalance in the

microbiota can contribute to constipation. Maintaining a diet rich in probiotics and prebiotics can help maintain a healthy microbiome.

### 46. What are prebiotics, and how can they help with constipation?

Prebiotics are types of fiber that feed beneficial bacteria in the gut. They can improve digestive health and help relieve constipation by increasing fecal bulk and improving intestinal motility.

### 47. What are probiotics, and how can they help with constipation?

Probiotics are live microorganisms that can improve intestinal health. Certain strains, such as Bifidobacterium and Lactobacillus, are effective in improving stool frequency and consistency in people with constipation.

### 48. What is fecal impaction, and how is it treated?

Fecal impaction is a severe condition where hard stool becomes trapped in the colon or rectum. It is a complication of chronic constipation and may require medical treatment, including laxatives, suppositories, enemas, or, in severe cases, manual removal by a healthcare professional.

### 49. What are enemas, and how are they used to treat constipation?

An enema is a procedure that introduces fluid into the rectum through the anus to stimulate a bowel movement. They are used as a short-term treatment for severe constipation, fecal impaction, or before specific medical procedures. They should not be used regularly without the guidance of a medical professional.

### 50. What foods help relieve constipation?

Foods rich in fiber, such as fruits (especially plums and apples), vegetables, legumes, whole grains, and nuts, can help relieve constipation. We will see this in the chapter "Food".

### 51. Are there specific foods that should be avoided if you suffer from constipation?

Some low-fiber or highly processed foods, such as white bread, sweets and processed meats, often worsen constipation. Focusing on a diet rich in fruits, vegetables, and whole grains is advisable. We will discuss this in detail in the "Food" chapter.

### 52. How does a high-protein diet influence constipation?

A diet high in protein but deficient in fiber can contribute to constipation. Therefore, balancing protein intake with sufficient fiber sources, such as fruits, vegetables, and whole grains, is essential.

### 53. How can the ketogenic diet affect constipation?

The ketogenic diet, which is low in carbohydrates and high in fat, can lead to lower fiber intake, which can result in constipation. Increasing the intake of fiber-rich vegetables and staying well-hydrated may help.

### 54. How does meal timing influence constipation?

Irregular meal times can affect the natural rhythm of the bowel. Eating at regular times can help synchronize the digestive process and improve bowel regularity.

### 55. How can exercise influence constipation?

Regular physical exercise stimulates the digestive system, increasing intestinal motility and facilitating the passage of stool through the colon. Walking, swimming, or practicing yoga can be especially beneficial.

### 56. Is high-intensity exercise beneficial for constipation?

Exercise in general, including high-intensity activities such as running or interval training, often stimulates bowel movements and helps relieve constipation.

### 57. Can magnesium supplements help with constipation?

Magnesium has a natural laxative effect, often helping many people relieve constipation by drawing water into the intestines and stimulating bowel movements. We will see this in the "Supplements" chapter.

### 58. What role does bowel position play in constipation?

Posture during bowel movements can influence the ease of

evacuation. Adopting a squatting position or elevating both feet with a stool can better align the rectum and facilitate stool passage.

### 59. How can natural oils, such as olive oil, help with constipation?

Consuming natural oils, such as olive or coconut oil, can act as lubricants in the intestines, facilitating the passage of stool. Taking a small amount on an empty stomach or adding a tablespoon of oil to the daily diet can help with constipation.

### 60. How does a vegan or vegetarian diet affect constipation?

Vegan or vegetarian diets, which are often rich in fiber, can help prevent constipation. However, it is essential to consume a variety of fiber-rich foods.

### 61. Can yoga relieve constipation?

Yoga can help improve digestion and relieve constipation by increasing circulation to the intestines and reducing stress. Specific postures are specifically designed to stimulate the digestive system.

### 62. What is acupuncture, and can it be helpful for constipation?

Acupuncture is a traditional Chinese medicine practice that involves inserting fine needles into specific points on the body. Some studies conclude that it can help improve bowel function and relieve constipation.

### 63. How can breastfeeding influence the baby's constipation?

Exclusively breastfed infants rarely experience constipation, as breast milk is easily digested and absorbed. However, if a formula is introduced, there may be a temporary change in bowel habits.

### 64. What is the gastrocolic reflex, and how is it related to constipation?

The gastrocolic reflex is a physiological response in which the intake of food stimulates the movement of the colon. Some people may not have this reflex functioning correctly, which can contribute to constipation. Eating regularly and maintaining a balanced diet can help stimulate this reflex.

### 65. How does travel or changes in routine affect constipation?

Travel or changes in routine may alter bowel habits due to changes in diet, stress and disruption of regular schedules, which may contribute to temporary constipation.

### 66. How important is routine in preventing constipation?

Changes in sleep schedule, diet, or physical activity can alter the natural rhythm of the bowel and contribute to constipation. Maintaining a balanced diet and good hydration can help mitigate these effects.

### 67. How can bathing habits influence constipation?

Establishing a regular toilet routine, preferably at the same time every day, and not ignoring the need for bowel movements can help promote bowel regularity and prevent constipation. Additionally, creating a relaxed and comfortable environment can help facilitate bowel movements.

### 68. Are there massage techniques that can relieve constipation?

Yes, gentle abdominal massage can help stimulate the bowels and promote stool movement. This approach can be effective in combination with other methods, such as a balanced diet and regular exercise.

### 69. Can herbal teas help with constipation?

Some herbal teas contain laxative properties that can help alleviate constipation. We will discuss this in the chapter on "Medicinal Plants."

### 70. What is a colonoscopy, and when is it recommended for constipation?

A colonoscopy is a procedure that enables physicians to examine the inside of the colon and rectum. In cases of chronic constipation, it is recommended to rule out obstructions, polyps, tumors, or inflammatory bowel diseases.

### 71. What is idiopathic chronic constipation?

Idiopathic chronic constipation is a form of constipation without an apparent medical cause. Difficult or infrequent bowel movements are characteristic of it and may require dietary and lifestyle adjustments, as well as natural or medical treatments in some cases.

### 72. Can irritable bowel syndrome cause constipation?

Yes, IBS can cause episodes of constipation alternating with diarrhea. Management of IBS often involves making dietary changes and focusing on stress management.

### 73. How can irritable bowel syndrome (IBS) with constipation be differentiated from other types of constipation?

IBS with constipation is accompanied by recurrent abdominal pain, bloating, and changes in the shape of the stool. Unlike functional constipation, IBS involves a combination of digestive symptoms and is often related to emotional and stress factors.

### 74. What is irritable bowel syndrome (IBS), and how is it related to constipation?

IBS is a functional gastrointestinal disorder characterized by abdominal pain and changes in bowel habits, including constipation. Treatment may include dietary adjustments, stress management techniques, and targeted supplements or medications.

### 75. What is the FODMAP diet, and how can it help with constipation?

The FODMAP diet is low in certain fermentable carbohydrates (fermentable oligosaccharides, disaccharides, monosaccharides and polyols), which can be challenging to digest and may contribute to intestinal problems. Although primarily used for irritable bowel syndrome, reducing certain FODMAPs may help relieve constipation in some people.

### 76. How does the low FODMAP diet influence constipation?

A low FODMAP diet may be helpful for some people with irritable bowel syndrome with constipation (IBS-E). Reducing certain fermentable carbohydrates may alleviate digestive symptoms, although this approach is not suitable for everyone.

### 77. What is biofeedback, and how can it help with constipation?

Biofeedback is a technique that teaches people to control specific bodily processes. For constipation, it can help retrain the pelvic floor muscles to improve the evacuation process. It can be helpful for people with pelvic floor dysfunction that causes constipation.

### 78. How can surgery affect constipation?

Some surgeries, especially those involving the abdomen, may temporarily affect bowel movement and cause postoperative constipation due to bowel manipulation and the use of opioid analgesics. Early motility, following dietary recommendations after surgery, and hydrating well can help mitigate this effect.

### 79. What is colectomy, and when is it considered for constipation?

A colonectomy is a surgery that removes part or all of the colon. It is considered in severe cases of chronic constipation that do not respond to other treatments, especially when there is a severe structural or functional problem in the colon.

### 80. What is pelvic floor dysfunction, and how is it related to constipation?

Pelvic floor dysfunction involves problems with the muscles and nerves that help control defecation. It can make it challenging to have a proper bowel movement, contributing to chronic constipation. Treatment may include physical therapy, Kegel exercises, or biofeedback.

### 81. What is dyssynergic defecation?

Dyssynergic defecation occurs when the pelvic floor muscles fail to relax adequately during bowel movements, making the process difficult. Biofeedback and pelvic physical therapy can be effective in treating this condition.

### 82. What is pelvic floor dyssynergia, and how is it related to constipation?

Pelvic floor dyssynergia occurs when the pelvic floor muscles fail to relax properly during bowel movements. This can make it challenging to have a bowel movement and contribute to the development of constipation.

### 83. What is an incomplete bowel movement, and how is it related to constipation?

The sensation of incomplete bowel movement is the feeling that the bowel has not been completely emptied after defecation. It is a common symptom in people with chronic constipation and may be related to motility problems or pelvic floor dysfunction.

### 84. How can neurological disorders affect constipation?

Neurological disorders such as multiple sclerosis, Parkinson's disease, spinal cord injury and stroke can affect bowel function by damaging the nerves that control the bowel, which can lead to constipation.

### 85. How does multiple sclerosis affect constipation?

Multiple sclerosis can affect the nerves that control the bowel, which can lead to constipation. Management may include a combination of a high-fiber diet, adequate hydration, physical activity and medications if necessary.

### 86. How does Parkinson's disease affect constipation?

Parkinson's disease can affect autonomic function, including bowel control. This can slow bowel transit and cause constipation. Treatment may include dietary changes, exercise, and, in some cases, specific supplements or medications to improve bowel motility.

### 87. What is colonic inertia, and how is it related to constipation?

Colonic inertia is a condition in which the colon moves slowly or is reduced in movement, resulting in severe constipation. Treatment may include dietary changes, supplements, medications that stimulate the bowel, or, in extreme cases, surgery.

### 88. What is slow colonic transit, and how is it related to constipation?

Slowed colonic transit is when stool moves more slowly than usual through the colon. This can result in chronic constipation. It can be treated with dietary changes, natural supplements, or medications, and, in severe cases, surgery may be necessary.

### 89. What is lazy bowel syndrome, and how is it treated?

Lazy bowel syndrome, also known as atonic or hypotonic bowel, refers to a colon that has lost its ability to contract efficiently, often due to the overuse of laxatives. This can result in chronic constipation. Treatment may include gradually reducing laxatives under the supervision of a healthcare professional, making dietary changes, and increasing physical activity.

### 90. How can psychological disorders affect constipation?

Psychological disorders such as depression and anxiety can affect bowel function and contribute to constipation. Treatment may include psychological therapy, stress management, physical activity, dietary changes, and, in some cases, supplementation or medication.

### 91. How is depression related to constipation?

Depression can influence bowel function due to changes in eating habits, physical activity and circadian rhythm. In addition, some antidepressants may have the side effect of constipation. Integrated treatment that addresses both mental health, dietary, and lifestyle changes may be necessary.

### 92. How can diabetes affect constipation?

Diabetes, mainly if not well controlled, can cause autonomic neuropathy, which affects the nerves that control the bowel, slowing bowel motility and contributing to constipation. Proper blood sugar control, exercise and an adequate fiber-rich diet can help mitigate this problem.

### 93. What is proctalgia fugax, and how is it related to constipation?

Proctalgia fugax is a brief, severe pain in the rectum that may occur sporadically. Although not directly caused by constipation, bowel difficulties may aggravate or trigger episodes in some people.

### 94. What is Ogilvie's syndrome, and how is it related to constipation?

Ogilvie's syndrome, also known as acute colonic pseudo-obstruction, is a massive dilatation of the colon without an apparent mechanical cause. It can cause severe constipation and abdominal distention and usually requires urgent medical attention.

### 95. How can hypercalcemia contribute to constipation?

Hypercalcemia, or elevated blood calcium levels, can cause constipation by affecting the function of the bowel muscles. To relieve symptoms, treating the underlying cause of hyper-calcemia is essential.

### 96. How does excessive calcium intake affect constipation?

Excessive intake of calcium supplements can cause constipation by reducing intestinal motility. The diet must balance calcium with sufficient magnesium and fiber to prevent this effect.

### 97. What is overlap syndrome, and how is it related to constipation?

Overlap syndrome refers to the simultaneous presence of more than one functional gastrointestinal disorder, such as IBS with constipation and functional dyspepsia. Symptoms may be more complex and require a multifaceted treatment approach.

### 98. What is a megacolon, and how is it related to constipation?

Megacolon is an abnormal dilation of the colon that can be either congenital or acquired. This condition can lead to severe constipation, as the dilated colon has difficulty moving stool efficiently.

### 99. How can short bowel syndrome affect constipation?

Short bowel syndrome occurs when a significant portion of the small intestine has been removed or is not functioning correctly. Although it often causes diarrhea, it can also lead to constipation due to imbalances in fluid and nutrient absorption.

### 100. What is the BRAT diet, and how can it influence constipation?

The BRAT (Bananas, Rice, Applesauce, Toast) diet is astringent and fiberless. If followed for a long time, constipation can worsen. However, it is most commonly used to treat diarrhea.

### 101. How can a low-residue diet help in cases of constipation?

A low-residue diet limits the amount of fiber and foods that leave residue in the colon, which may be helpful in some instances of constipation related to blockages or inflammation. However, a high-fiber diet is generally more beneficial for constipation in the long term.

### 102. How can inflammatory bowel diseases affect constipation?

Although inflammatory bowel diseases, such as Crohn's disease and ulcerative colitis, often cause diarrhea, they can also cause constipation due to inflammation or narrowing of the bowel. Treatment focuses on controlling the inflammation.

### 103. What is obstructed defecation syndrome, and how is it treated?

Obstructed defecation syndrome is difficulty in passing stool due to functional or anatomical problems in the rectum or pelvic floor. Treatment may include biofeedback, physical therapy, or surgery in severe cases.

### 104. What is intestinal obstruction, and how is it different from constipation?

Intestinal obstruction is a physical blockage in the intestine that prevents the passage of stool. Although more intense, it can cause symptoms similar to constipation, such as abdominal pain and lack of bowel movements. It is a medical emergency that requires immediate attention. Conversely, constipation is difficulty passing stools due to hard stools or slow bowel movements.

**105. How does malnutrition affect constipation?**
Malnutrition, particularly a deficiency in fiber and fluids in the diet, can contribute to constipation. Ensuring adequate intake of essential nutrients is crucial to maintaining healthy bowel function.

**106. How does fibromyalgia affect constipation?**
Fibromyalgia may be associated with irritable bowel syndrome, including the constipation-predominant subtype. Pain management, stress, and diet are key components of treatment.

**107. How can chemotherapy affect constipation?**
Chemotherapy, which affects the gastrointestinal tract and reduces intestinal motility, may cause constipation. Pain medications used during treatment may also contribute to the condition. Management includes hydration, a balanced diet, and the use of laxatives as needed.

**108. What are glycerin suppositories, and how do they help with constipation?**
Glycerin suppositories are a type of rectal laxative that helps stimulate bowel movement by gently irritating the lining of the rectum. They are effective in relieving occasional constipation.

**109. What is colonic cleansing, and is it recommended for constipation?**
Colonic cleansing involves flushing the colon with large amounts of water. It is not recommended as a treatment for constipation, as it can cause electrolyte imbalances and damage the intestinal flora.

# SUGGESTED PRACTICAL PLAN

Here, you'll find a comprehensive and detailed guide to help you manage constipation and effectively alleviate its symptoms. This holistic approach not only helps you feel relief but also acts as an essential first step toward reclaiming your overall well-being. Now is the perfect time to prioritize your health and start living more comfortably!

▸ **Discover the Causes**: Identifying the root cause of constipation is crucial for effective treatment. Understanding the potential triggers and addressing them can make a significant difference in your recovery process. To help with this, I recommend exploring the chapter "Constipation", especially the sections "Causes" and "Symptom Relief and Prevention". There, you'll find practical tools and clear guidance to pinpoint and reduce the underlying triggers effectively.

▸ **Add Nutritional Supplements**: Enhance your recovery by incorporating nutritional supplements into your daily routine. These supplements can be the perfect complement to your diet, contributing significantly to your treatment's success. In the next chapter, you'll discover safe, natural, and effective options that can boost your digestive health and overall well-being.

▸ **Discover the Benefits of Herbal Medicine**: Herbal medicine, which harnesses the power of medicinal plants, can be an excellent ally in managing constipation. In the chapter "Medicinal Plants", you'll find a thorough guide to the best natural solutions, paired with practical recipes to provide quick and effective relief, all while maintaining your body's natural balance.

▸ **Diet to Combat Constipation**: Your diet plays a fundamental role in the health of your digestive system. Certain foods can be your strongest allies, while others might exacerbate the issue. In the chapters "Foods That Transform" and "Juices and Smoothies", you'll discover detailed, practical insights, along with over 50 delicious recipes and a curated selection of juices specifically designed to ease constipation. Adopting a gut-friendly diet has never been so easy—or so enjoyable.

▸ **Identify Potential Allergens**: Foods like gluten, dairy, or even pork might negatively impact your digestive system without you realizing it. Consider eliminating them temporarily from your diet for at least two weeks and then gradually reintroducing them, one at a time, to observe how your body responds. These small dietary experiments could lead to remarkable improvements in your quality of life.

▸ **Review Your Medications**: If you suspect that any medications you are taking (for constipation or other conditions) might be contributing to the problem, it's essential to discuss this with your doctor. Never stop a medication on your own, as doing so could harm your health. However, your doctor can evaluate the situation, adjust dosages, or recommend alternatives to minimize side effects and support your recovery. Remember, your health and well-being should always come first.

▸ **Lifestyle Changes**: Your everyday habits play a significant role in your digestive health, and making small adjustments can help relieve constipation. In the chapter "Symptom Relief and Prevention", you'll find actionable recommendations to help you make simple changes that can significantly improve your comfort and well-being.

▸ **Include Exercise in Your Routine**: Physical activity is essential for maintaining intestinal health. Regular exercise, even if it's just walking for 20-30 minutes a day, can stimulate bowel movements, improve intestinal function, and reduce the discomfort associated with constipation.

▸ **The Importance of Hydration**: Proper hydration is vital to the healthy functioning of your digestive system. Aim to drink at least six glasses of water daily, and increase this to eight if you engage in physical activity. These small lifestyle changes, like staying hydrated, can make a noticeable difference in your overall health and comfort.

## Are You Facing Other Related Issues?

If, in addition to constipation, you're dealing with conditions like hemorrhoids, varicose veins, or SIBO (Small Intestinal Bacterial Overgrowth), I invite you to explore some of my other books. These resources offer practical advice and natural solutions tailored to these specific issues:

▸ **HEMORRHOIDS**. Foods, Supplements & Herbs
▸ **SIBO**. Foods, Supplements & Herbs
▸ **VARICOSE VEINS**. Foods, Supplements & Herbs

These complementary guides are designed to help you understand these conditions more fully and enhance your quality of life with practical, natural strategies.

Start Your Journey to Better Health Today!

# NUTRITIONAL SUPPLEMENTS

*"Proper nutrition is the key to a healthy and active life" (Albert Einstein)*

Nutritional supplements have become a valuable ally in the pursuit of better health and an enhanced quality of life. These options–available in various user-friendly formats such as tablets, capsules, powders, or easily consumable liquids–are purposefully designed to complement your daily nutrition by delivering essential nutrients that can be challenging to obtain through regular meals alone. Packed with powerful components like vitamins, minerals, amino acids, antioxidants, and other bioactive compounds, these supplements are expertly formulated in precise proportions to meet the unique needs of every individual–even when the demands are high. Whether you're navigating restrictive diets, facing nutritional gaps, or coping with increased physical or mental demands, supplements can provide the extra support your body needs.

Beyond simply filling in nutritional gaps, supplements offer an array of tailored benefits to suit diverse lifestyles and health challenges. They can help boost energy, improve physical performance, support those managing fast-paced lives, and provide practical solutions for staying balanced and resilient. Their significance often becomes even more apparent during times of illness, specific health conditions, or chronic issues. In these situations, supplements do more than complement a diet–they can actively help restore altered functions, ease symptoms, and assist in more complex recovery processes. They serve as companions in the pursuit of health, helping you sustain and rebuild your vitality.

Effectively integrating supplements into your routine requires thoughtful use grounded in science and, when needed, professional guidance. By understanding their benefits and approaching them with care, supplements can evolve into powerful tools for improving your overall well-being in a sustainable and meaningful way. Remember–every step you take toward caring for your body is a step closer to feeling stronger, more energized, and more capable of facing life's challenges with confidence.

Take that step today. Your path to better health begins with small but impactful choices!

## Essential Precautions

Understanding the risks associated with supplements is vital, as they can sometimes cause side effects, have contraindications, or interact with medications. It's important to thoroughly review the potential adverse effects detailed at the end of this chapter. Take a moment to assess your overall health and avoid any supplements that could conflict with the medications you're currently taking or exacerbate existing medical conditions. Prioritizing this step ensures a safer and more effective approach to improving your well-being.

## Nutritional Supplements and Constipation

In the journey toward optimal health and well-being, maintaining a healthy digestive system plays a vital role. Yet, for many people, constipation remains a frustrating and often isolating challenge. This condition goes beyond physical discomfort, creating an emotional toll that can significantly impact everyday life and overall happiness.

The good news is that scientific advancements in recent years have shed light on natural, accessible, and effective ways to manage constipation. Nutritional supplements have emerged as powerful allies in restoring healthy bowel regularity and promoting long-term gastrointestinal balance. From soluble fibers to probiotics and digestive enzymes, these supplements have gained recognition for their ability to gently support the body's natural processes while improving digestive comfort.

In the sections ahead, we'll dive into the most effective

nutritional supplements for constipation, highlighting their benefits and recommended average dosages. You'll find this guide conveniently organized alphabetically, making it easy to explore which options might be the perfect fit for your needs. Let's take the first step toward relief and reclaiming your digestive health!

# Castor Oil

Castor oil is known for its natural laxative properties and has been traditionally used as a remedy to relieve constipation. Below, I will mention some of the benefits of castor oil for this problem, as well as the average recommended dosage:

▸ Natural laxative: It contains a compound called ricinoleic acid, which acts as a mild laxative. This acid stimulates receptors in the intestine's lining, promoting bowel movements and helping relieve constipation.

▸ Facilitates waste elimination: Helps soften the stool, making it easier to pass through the intestine. This can be especially useful in cases of chronic constipation or when stools are hard and challenging to pass.

▸ Stimulates bowel function: Castor oil acts as a laxative, helping to stimulate muscle activity and encourage a regular bowel rhythm, thereby promoting waste evacuation.

**Recommended average dosage:**
Although it may vary according to the age and condition of the individual, the average recommended dosage is as follows:

The recommended dose is 15 to 60 ml of castor oil, taken daily before bedtime. However, you can start with a low dose and gradually increase it according to your body's response.

# Chia

Chia seeds are a food rich in fiber and nutrients, offering several benefits that can help relieve constipation. Here are a few of them:

▸ High fiber content: Chia seeds are an excellent source of both soluble and insoluble fiber. Insoluble fiber helps increase stool bulk, soften stool, and facilitate its passage through the intestine. Soluble fiber, on the other hand, absorbs water and forms a gel that helps maintain proper stool consistency.

▸ Promotes bowel regularity: Chia seeds' high fiber content helps regularize bowel movements and prevent constipation. Fiber adds bulk to the stool and stimulates peristalsis, facilitating expulsion.

▸ Intestinal hydration: They can absorb up to 10 times their weight in water. When consumed, they form a gel in the intestine that helps maintain proper stool hydration, contributing to smoother and less painful bowel movements.

**Recommended average dosage:**
The recommended dose of chia seeds for constipation is 1 to 2 tablespoons per day. To allow the body to adjust to the additional fiber, it is recommended to start with a smaller amount and increase gradually. Chia seeds can be added to a variety of foods and beverages, including smoothies, yogurt, salads, and cereal.

Remember that consuming enough liquid when ingesting chia seeds is essential, as they absorb water.


# Magnesium Carbonate

Magnesium carbonate is commonly used to relieve constipation. Below, I will mention some of the benefits of this problem, as well as the average recommended dosage:

▸ Mild laxative: Magnesium carbonate acts as a mild laxative by drawing water into the intestine and increasing the water content of the stool. This property helps soften the stool and facilitates its passage through the intestine, thus relieving constipation.

▸ Stimulates bowel movements: Magnesium carbonate

promotes movement, helping maintain a healthy bowel rhythm and preventing constipation.

‣ Relieves abdominal discomfort: Constipation is often associated with discomfort and bloating. Magnesium carbonate helps alleviate these symptoms by promoting regular bowel movements and reducing abdominal pressure.

**Recommended average dosage:**
The typical dose of magnesium carbonate for constipation is 2 to 4 grams – approximately 1/2 to 1 teaspoon – mixed with water.

It is usually most effective to take the maximum dose recommended by the manufacturer just before sleep. However, you can take it one or two hours before or after meals and/or other treatments. You can take it right after eating if you experience digestive discomfort on an empty stomach.

# Probiotics

Probiotics are beneficial microorganisms naturally found in the digestive system and can provide several benefits to relieve constipation. Here are a few of them:

‣ Restoration of intestinal balance: Probiotics help to restore and maintain a healthy balance of bacteria in the gut. This is especially relevant when constipation is associated with intestinal dysbiosis, i.e., an alteration in the composition of the intestinal microbiota.

‣ Improved intestinal motility: Certain probiotic strains, such as Bifidobacterium lactis and Lactobacillus acidophilus, have been demonstrated to enhance intestinal motility. These probiotics may also stimulate regular bowel movements and help prevent constipation.

‣ Increased production of short-chain fatty acids: Probiotics can ferment undigested waste in the intestine and produce short-chain fatty acids, such as butyrate. These fatty acids enhance intestinal function, increase stool hydration, and promote regularity in the intestines.

**Recommended dosage:**
The recommended dosage may vary depending on the type of probiotic strain and individual needs. It is typically between 1 and 10 billion colony-forming units (CFU) daily. Follow the manufacturer's instructions.

**Posology:**
It is recommended to be taken in the morning or at night. Follow the manufacturer's directions.

**Average action time:**
Although the onset of action may vary, it usually shows beneficial effects on digestive health and gut microbiota balance after a few weeks of continuous use.

**Maximum recommended time of continuous use:**
There is no established maximum time for continuous use, as they are safe for consumption for more than six months. To maintain intestinal health, it is recommended to follow the manufacturer's directions or consult a specialist if side effects occur or if you plan to use them for more than six months consecutively.

# Psyllium

Psyllium seeds are a dietary supplement commonly used to treat constipation. Some of its benefits are listed below:

▸ Promotes bowel regularity: Psyllium fiber is a source of soluble fiber that absorbs water in the intestine, forming a gelatinous mass that facilitates the passage of stool. This effect increases stool bulk and stimulates bowel regularity, relieving constipation.

▸ Improves stool consistency: Psyllium fiber also helps improve stool consistency. If stools are too complex and dry, adding moisture and softness makes them easier to pass.

‣ Relieves abdominal discomfort: Constipation often leads to abdominal pain and bloating. Psyllium fiber helps alleviate these symptoms by promoting regular bowel movements and reducing abdominal pressure.

**Recommended average dosage:**
The typical dose of psyllium fiber is 5 to 10 grams once or twice daily. It is recommended that psyllium fiber be mixed with water or another liquid and consumed immediately. Gradually increasing the dose is essential to allow the body to adjust and avoid possible side effects, such as bloating or gas.

# Rhubarb

Rhubarb root has been traditionally used as a natural remedy to relieve constipation. Here are some of the benefits:

‣ Laxative effect: Rhubarb root contains natural compounds, such as emodin and anthraquinone, which have laxative properties. These compounds stimulate and promote regular bowel movements, thus relieving constipation.

‣ Stimulates bile secretion: Increases bile production and secretion in the liver, improving digestion and intestinal transit. Better digestion can help prevent constipation and promote regular bowel movements.

‣ Improves intestinal motility: It stimulates contractions in the intestine, helping to move stool and prevent constipation.

**Recommended average dosage:**
The typical dose of rhubarb root for adults with constipation is 0.5 to 1 gram daily. It is recommended to take it before bedtime for a morning laxative effect. Staying within the recommended dose and following the product's specific directions is essential.

## Adverse Effects, Contraindications, and Interactions

This is essential information regarding the potential side effects, contraindications, and interactions of the recommended supplements. Please read it thoroughly and carefully before taking any of them to ensure your safety and optimal use.

## Castor Oil

▸ **Side effects**: It may cause diarrhea, abdominal cramps and nausea. If not enough liquid is consumed, it may also cause dehydration.

▸ **Contraindications**: It is not recommended for use in pregnant women due to its potential to stimulate uterine contractions. It should also be avoided in people with intestinal obstruction, inflammatory bowel disease, appendicitis, kidney, or liver problems.

▸ **Interactions**: Castor oil may interact with blood-thinning medications, antidiabetic drugs, non-steroidal anti-inflammatory drugs and other laxatives. If you are taking any of these medications, it is essential to consult a physician before using castor oil.

## Magnesium Carbonate

▸ **Side effects**: It may cause diarrhea, nausea, vomiting and stomach upset. It may also have a laxative effect.

▸ **Contraindications**: It is not recommended for people with renal insufficiency, heart disease, intestinal obstruction, or elevated blood magnesium levels.

▸ **Interactions**: It may interact with antibiotics, heart medications, and osteoporosis medications. If you are taking any medication, it is essential to consult your doctor.

## Chia Seeds

▸ **Side effects**: Chia seeds are generally well-tolerated, but some people may experience gas, abdominal bloating, or digestive problems when consuming them in large quantities or without sufficient liquid.

▸ **Contraindications**: No significant contraindications have been reported for the consumption of chia seeds. However, because they can expand in the stomach, they should be consumed in moderation and accompanied by liquid.

▸ **Interactions**: No significant interactions of chia seeds with medications have been reported. However, it is essential to consult a physician if you are taking any medicines to evaluate possible interactions.

## Psyllium Fiber

▸ **Side effects**: Some people may experience gas, bloating, or diarrhea when taking psyllium fiber. It is essential to start with low doses and increase gradually to allow the body to adapt.

▸ **Contraindications**: This treatment may not be suitable for people with narrowing of the esophagus or intestinal tract, or for those experiencing difficulty swallowing.

▸ **Interactions**: Psyllium fiber may affect drug absorption, so it is recommended to take it at least two hours before or after taking medications. You should consult your doctor to evaluate potential interactions if you are taking medications.

## Probiotics

▸ **Side effects**: Probiotics are generally considered safe; however, some people may experience gas, abdominal bloating, or diarrhea. These side effects are typically temporary and usually disappear as the body adjusts.

▸ **Contraindications**: Not recommended for people with weakened immune systems or those with intravenous catheters.

▸ **Interactions**: It may interact with certain medications, including antibiotics and immunosuppressive drugs. If you are taking any medications, consult your doctor.

## Rhubarb

▸ **Side Effects**: Excessive consumption of rhubarb root may cause diarrhea, abdominal cramps, nausea and vomiting. It may also produce a reddish color in the urine.

▸ **Contraindications**: Its use is not recommended in people with intestinal obstruction, inflammatory bowel disease, appendicitis, or kidney or liver problems. It should also be avoided during pregnancy and lactation.

▸ **Interactions**: Rhubarb root may interfere with the absorption of certain medications, including blood thinners, diuretics, and cardiovascular drugs. If you are taking any of these medications, it is essential to consult a physician before using rhubarb root.

# FOODS THAT TRANSFORM

*"The doctor of the future will not treat the human body with drugs, but will prevent disease with nutrition" (Thomas Edison)*

Throughout history, our diet has undergone profoundly radical changes, sharply diverging from the habits of our ancestors. Millions of years ago, early humans shaped their diet around what they could gather or hunt, relying on fresh and raw foods provided by their environment. The emergence of agriculture and livestock farming marked the beginning of a new era of human nutrition, further accelerated by the Industrial Revolution. However, it is important to recognize that while our dietary habits have evolved drastically, our genetics have remained virtually unchanged.

Over time, foods such as dairy products, grains, refined sugars, and vegetable oils were introduced, alongside the rise of intensive meat production. These innovations have made meals more accessible and convenient, yet they have also led to significant changes in nutritional composition. Furthermore, advances in food preservation and culinary techniques gave rise to new methods of storage and preparation, which inevitably impacted food quality.

In recent years, an alarming trend has surfaced: modern diets have become dominated by ultra-processed foods, contributing to the widespread increase in chronic illnesses. Conditions such as obesity, type 2 diabetes, hypertension, and a variety of cardiovascular and digestive disorders have all been closely linked to this dietary shift. Why is this happening? Primarily because ultra-processed foods are heavily laden with refined carbohydrates, unhealthy fats, added sugars, chemical additives, and low-quality vegetable oils. Even meats and other animal products from intensive farming systems are often filled with substances harmful to health. These processed foods have largely replaced traditional diets, which were built on fresh and natural ingredients, disrupting the equilibrium that once fostered optimal well-being among our ancestors.

Nonetheless, there is hope for reversing this trend: small yet thoughtful changes to our eating habits can have a significant impact on our health. Returning to a balanced, nutrient-rich way of eating, centered on fresh, whole foods, is essential for establishing a strong foundation for wellness. Integrating fruits, vegetables, root vegetables, legumes, nuts, and seeds into the diet is a powerful step toward revitalizing the way we nourish ourselves. Despite this, one major challenge persists: the consumption of these natural, unprocessed foods remains astonishingly low in many parts of the world.

Choosing a lifestyle rooted in mindful eating not only helps prevent diseases associated with poor dietary habits but also rejuvenates the body and mind. By prioritizing real, wholesome foods and cutting back on ultra-processed options, we can cultivate a healthier, more balanced, and fulfilling life. Now is the time to rediscover the transformative power of a healthy diet—not as a form of restriction, but as an act of self-care. Your health deserves that commitment!

## Understanding the Link Between Nutrition and Health

How often have you asked yourself if what you eat truly supports your well-being? The relationship between nutrition and health is far deeper than we commonly realize. Understanding which foods promote wellness and which ones to avoid, tailored to your specific needs, is a powerful step toward improving your quality of life. This isn't a new concept; it has been examined and revered for centuries. Since ancient times, cultures around the world have recognized the therapeutic value of nutrition as a means to heal, strengthen, and sustain the body, leaving us a profound legacy of wisdom.

Traditional medical systems—such as Traditional Chinese Medicine, the practices of ancient Egypt, Greece, and Rome,

Ayurveda in India, and indigenous healing methods across the Americas–delved into the restorative potential of natural foods. These practices emphasized the idea that food does much more than nourish; it can protect, alleviate discomfort, and even heal the body.

For many years, these age-old principles were often dismissed by conventional medicine as unscientific. Yet, modern research has gradually confirmed what our ancestors intuitively understood: the foods we eat directly affect not only our physical health but also our emotional well-being. Today, scientific studies continue to uncover compounds in food with therapeutic properties that help prevent diseases, reduce symptoms, and promote overall health.

Researchers have spent decades analyzing how certain foods strengthen the body and protect against chronic illnesses, identifying dietary patterns in populations with low disease rates that differ significantly from those in less healthy communities. These studies reveal the decisive role specific nutrients play in promoting vitality and longevity, with certain foods offering unique benefits such as anti-inflammatory properties to manage joint pain and chronic discomfort, antimicrobial effects to bolster immune defenses, anticoagulant actions to support cardiovascular health, antihypertensive abilities to regulate blood pressure, and mood-enhancing compounds that alleviate anxiety while fostering emotional resilience.

What you choose to eat influences not only your daily energy but also your capacity to recover, fend off illness, and pursue a fulfilling life. On the flip side, a poor diet or reliance on unhealthy foods can exacerbate health problems, intensify symptoms, and undermine overall well-being.

The encouraging part? Every day offers the chance to make dietary choices that lead to better health. While external factors like pollution or environmental changes may remain out of your control, your diet is a fundamental tool for self-care. Each ingredient on your plate carries the potential to positively impact both your physical and mental health.

Learning which foods are best for your unique needs–and understanding which ones may harm your health–can empower you to find balance and achieve a healthier, more vibrant lifestyle. Nutrition, humanity's earliest form of medicine, is not just a pathway to wellness but also a connection to our roots, equipping us for a future filled with possibilities.

I invite you to explore how nutrition can become your strongest ally in easing ailments, building resilience, and fostering happiness. Are you ready to embrace this journey of discovery and transformation? Your well-being is within your control, and every meal is a chance to create a life of greater health and vitality.

Start today: Nourish your body, refresh your mind, and live fully.

## Cooking Techniques

Healthy cooking is essential for everyone, especially after the age of 40. Below are various cooking techniques along with their related health benefits and potential risks.

### Healthier Ways of Cooking

▸ **Steaming**: Steaming is an excellent method for preserving nutrients, as it does not require the use of additional fats. It helps keep food tender and juicy while being a gentle cooking technique that does not contribute to the formation of harmful compounds.

▸ **Oven roasting**: Oven roasting is a healthy option that does not require added oils. Foods like vegetables, fish, and chicken can be roasted in the oven to create nutritious and flavorful meals.

▸ **Light sautéing**: This method involves quickly cooking food over high heat with a small amount of healthy oil, such as olive or coconut oil. Light sautéing helps maintain the food's texture and nutrients while cooking it efficiently.

▸ **Boiling**: Boiling is a healthy cooking method, particularly for vegetables. It preserves nutrients and creates a tender texture. However, it is crucial to avoid overcooking to minimize nutrient loss.

▸ **Baking**: Baking is an excellent way to prepare food without the need for added oils. Foods like fish, poultry, vegetables, and whole grains can be baked for healthy and flavorful dishes.

## Less Healthy Ways of Cooking

▸ **Frying**: Frying involves submerging food in hot oil, which significantly increases its saturated fat and calorie content. Additionally, frying at high temperatures can produce harmful compounds that pose health risks.

▸ **Breading and battering**: Coating food in breading or batter increases its calorie and fat content. These coatings can absorb more oil during cooking, resulting in a less nutritious meal.

▸ **Creamy sauces and dressings**: Cream-based sauces and dressings often contain high levels of saturated fat and excess calories. These can contribute to inflammation and exacerbate pain.

▸ **Grilling at high temperatures**: Cooking food on the grill at high heat can generate harmful compounds, such as polycyclic aromatic hydrocarbons (PAHs) and heterocyclic amines (HCAs), which have been associated with an increased cancer risk. Additionally, grilled meats can produce inflammatory substances.

Remember, the way you cook food significantly impacts its nutritional value and its overall effects on your health. Choosing healthy cooking methods ensures you maximize the benefits of your meals while reducing potential negative effects.

# Healing Foods According to TCM

In Traditional Chinese Medicine (TCM), food is considered a powerful therapeutic tool for restoring balance to the body and addressing specific health concerns, such as constipation. Below is a list of foods recommended in TCM to help with constipation and support overall well-being.

The most effective fruits with natural laxative properties include prunes, figs, oranges, apricots, and grapes. Additional foods that can aid in promoting digestive health include the following:

## Aloe Vera

The ideal is to use the pure gel extracted from the plant, but keep in mind that it is more concentrated than the prepared juice sold, so do not use more than 2 tablespoons. Mix 2 tablespoons of pure gel with the juice of some fruit and take it in the morning. Note: Use caution, as it may cause diarrhea in some people.

## Apple

Peel and thoroughly chew a raw apple about an hour after eating.

## Banana

Two ripe bananas between meals help relieve constipation.

## Carrot

If you suffer from chronic constipation, you should consume grated raw carrots daily, supplemented with 1 liter of carrot juice.

Recipe No. 2. Ingredients: 500 g of carrots and honey. Mash the carrot and add the honey to the juice. Mix well, and drink this preparation once in the morning and at night.

*Cautions*: Vinegar should not be added to carrots, as it may destroy their components. Additionally, as carotene is a soluble fat, it should be cooked with oil or another type of fat to prevent oxidation. Eating raw or cooked in water hinders the assimilation of carotene and causes it to lose its properties.

Other beneficial foods are papaya*, pumpkin, sesame and raw

almonds.

*Important note*: Pregnant women should not eat papaya, as it contains natural estrogens that could cause contractions and a risk of miscarriage. Additionally, pepsin and papain may impede the development of the fetus.

# Fig

Figs, whether fresh or dried, help cleanse the intestines of mucus and toxic waste, and also serve as a natural laxative.

# Flax Seeds

Mix 1 tablespoon of flax seeds in a glass of water, let it stand for at least 3 hours, and drink it before bed.

# Grape

Grapes or their juice are very effective. You can drink the juice on an empty stomach in the morning. Drinking one full glass per day is recommended until you see the effect. It is also highly recommended for children.

*Precautions*: According to TCM, as it contains an abundance of sugars, excessive ingestion may cause diarrhea, restlessness, and obnubilation (confusion, clumsiness of movement, psychic slowness, and decreased attention and perception).

# Honey

Dilute a tablespoon of honey in a glass of hot water and drink it on an empty stomach.

# Honey and Vinegar

Put 1 tablespoon of honey and 1 tablespoon of apple cider vinegar in a glass of water, mix well, and drink every 8 hours.

# Kiwifruit

Take two kiwis at breakfast. Precautions: According to TCM, kiwis can cause diarrhea due to their cold nature, so they should not be consumed excessively. They are especially discouraged for people predisposed to diarrhea or with delicate stomachs.

## Lemon

A glass of warm water with a teaspoon of freshly squeezed lemon juice and a pinch of salt on an empty stomach in the morning will help cleanse your intestines. Another remedy is to drink 2-3 glasses of warm water with lemon juice twice or three times a day.

## Molasses

Take 2 teaspoons in warm water 2 times a day.

## Olive Oil

Mix 1 tablespoon of olive oil with 1 teaspoon of lemon juice and drink it regularly.

## Peach

Eat 1 or 2 peaches about an hour after meals.

## Pineapple

Drink pineapple juice daily on an empty stomach until your intestines are regularized.

## Plum

Drink a glass of prune juice in the morning and another at night for immediate relief.

## Plums (dried)

Soak the dried plums the night before and drink both the water and the plums on an empty stomach.

## Raisins or Dried Grapes

Eat a handful a day, at least 1 hour after eating. You can also soak a handful of raisins in water overnight and then eat them on an empty stomach.

## Sodium Bicarbonate

Mix 1 teaspoon of baking soda in one-fourth cup of warm

water.

## Spinach

Raw spinach is the best natural remedy for irritated and sluggish intestines. You can eat it either raw or cooked. Precautions: According to Traditional Chinese Medicine (TCM), people experiencing stomach problems or diarrhea should consume it in small amounts. Additionally, since spinach contains oxalic acid, consuming it with calcium-rich foods, such as legumes, can form calcium oxalate, which hinders digestion and calcium absorption.

# Other Effective Remedies for Constipation

In addition to the recommended foods, there are various natural remedies and lifestyle changes that can effectively help relieve constipation:

▸ **Psyllium, Flax, or Linseed Seeds**
Preparation:
  - Soak 1 to 2 tablespoons of seeds in water or a plant-based drink (such as oat, almond, or soy milk) for several hours.
  - Before bedtime, drink both the liquid and the soaked seeds on an empty stomach.

These seeds are packed with fiber and mucilage, which help soften stools, improve intestinal transit, and facilitate bowel movements.

▸ **Warm Water with Honey on an Empty Stomach**
How to Use:
  - In the morning, drink a glass of warm water mixed with one tablespoon of honey on an empty stomach.
  - This remedy gently stimulates the digestive system, hydrates the intestines, and promotes the smooth passage of waste.

▸ **Extra Virgin Coconut Oil**
Instructions:
  - Take one tablespoon of extra virgin coconut oil before each main meal (breakfast, lunch, and dinner).
  - This oil not only supports intestinal motility but may also assist with weight management due to its healthy fats.

- Note: There's no need to worry about weight gain when consuming this oil in moderation, as it is unlikely to pose any issues.

### ‣ Hydration and Fiber Intake

Hydration: Drink at least 1.5 to 2 liters of water daily to ensure you stay hydrated. Proper hydration is essential for fiber to work effectively in the digestive system.

Increase Fiber-Rich Foods: Incorporate the following foods into your diet:
- Fresh fruits (e.g., apples, pears with their skin, or apricots).
- Vegetables (e.g., pumpkin, spinach, broccoli).
- Whole grains (e.g., oatmeal, brown rice, or whole-grain bread).

### Additional Recommendations
- Stay Active: Engage in daily physical activity, such as walking or light exercise, to stimulate intestinal movement.
- Establish a Routine: Set a regular schedule for going to the bathroom, ideally at the same time every day (such as after meals), to take advantage of the body's natural reflexes.

## General Dietary Recommendations

Diet plays a crucial role in both the prevention and management of constipation. Following a balanced diet that is rich in fiber and designed to support the optimal function of the digestive system is essential for improving bowel movement and maintaining overall health. Below are dietary recommendations to help you adjust your eating habits and effectively address this issue.

‣ **Increase your fiber intake**: Fiber is essential for preventing and treating constipation. Consuming at least 25-30 grams of fiber per day is recommended. Gradually increase your diet's fiber to allow your body to adjust. Include vegetables, fruits and legumes. Ideally, consume 3 to 5 servings of vegetables and 2 to 4 servings of fruits daily. However, it is advisable to consume fruit on an empty stomach, for example, half an hour before eating, and never during or at the end of a meal, as it causes gas and intestinal discomfort for many people.

▸ **Drink plenty of water**: Dehydration often worsens constipation, so it is essential to stay hydrated. Drink a considerable amount, 2 to 3 liters daily, but avoid drinking during meals. During meals, drink no more than half a glass of water. Non-carbonated water is preferable.

▸ **Eat regularly and avoid skipping meals**: Establishing regular meal times and refraining from skipping meals can help maintain your bowel rhythm. Try to eat at about the same time every day to establish a regular bowel movement pattern.

▸ **Eat balanced meals**: Include a variety of food groups in your daily meals, such as lean proteins (chicken, fish, legumes), whole grains (brown rice, quinoa, oatmeal), fruits, and vegetables. A balanced and varied diet provides the nutrients necessary for a healthy digestive system.

▸ **Limit processed and refined foods**: Processed and refined foods, such as baked goods made with white flour, fried foods and sweets, are often low in fiber and can exacerbate constipation. Opt for more natural and less processed foods to ensure you get enough fiber in your diet.

▸ **Get regular physical activity**: Regular exercise can help stimulate bowel movements and prevent constipation. Try getting at least 30 minutes of moderate physical activity daily, such as walking, swimming, or yoga.

▸ **Avoid stress**: Stress can impact the digestive system's functioning and contribute to constipation. Find ways to manage stress, such as practicing relaxation techniques, meditation, or engaging in physical activity. It is also essential to ensure that you have enough time to use the bathroom without feeling rushed or pressured.

▸ **Consider fiber supplements**: If your diet does not provide enough fiber, consider taking fiber supplements, such as psyllium, under the guidance of a healthcare professional. However, drinking enough water when taking fiber supplements is essential to avoid digestive discomfort.

▸ **Incorporate probiotic-rich foods**: Probiotics are healthy bacteria that help improve intestinal health and regularity of bowel transit. Probiotic-rich foods include plain yogurt, kefir, sauerkraut, kimchi and other fermented foods. Be sure to choose options with no added sugar for maximum benefits.

▸ **Please don't overdo it with foods that can cause constipation**: Some foods can have constipating effects in some people. These foods include white rice, cheese, green bananas, black tea and red meat. If you notice that any of these foods are affecting your bowel regularity, consider cutting back or seeking alternatives.

▸ **Avoid foods that irritate the bowel**: Some people may be sensitive to certain foods that can irritate the bowel, aggravating constipation. These foods may include spicy, fatty, high-caffeine, and high-sugar foods. Watch how your body reacts to these foods, and consider limiting your consumption if they worsen your symptoms.

▸ **Chew your food well**: Proper chewing is crucial for digestion and intestinal transit. Take time to chew each bite before swallowing. This helps break down food into smaller particles, facilitating its passage through the digestive system.

▸ **Avoid excessive alcohol consumption**: Alcohol can dehydrate the body and affect bowel function. Limit your alcohol intake and drink enough water to maintain good hydration.

▸ **Track your diet and symptoms**: Tracking your diet and symptoms can help you identify possible triggers for constipation. Write down what you eat and drink daily and any changes in your bowel habits. This will help you identify patterns and adjust your diet as needed.

▸ **Following a juice fast for several days** can be very helpful. The chapter "Juices & Smoothies" contains effective recipes for constipation.

Remember, each person is unique and may respond differently to specific foods and dietary changes.

## Recommended Food and Beverages

Here's a carefully curated selection of foods and beverages that can be especially effective in alleviating constipation and supporting healthy bowel movements. Adding these to your daily diet can significantly enhance your digestive well-being.

▸ **Foods rich in fiber**: Fiber is essential for maintaining good digestive health and preventing constipation. Fiber-rich foods help increase stool bulk and improve bowel transit. Some fiber-rich food choices include:

- *Fresh fruits*: Apples, pears, plums, oranges, raspberries, strawberries and blackberries are excellent choices due to their fiber and water content.

- *Vegetables*: Broccoli, spinach, carrots, zucchini, chard and kale are good sources of fiber, which helps prevent constipation.

- *Legumes*: Beans, lentils, chickpeas and peas are fiber-rich and provide vegetable protein.

- *Whole grains*: Brown rice, quinoa, oats and buckwheat are healthy choices that help improve constipation.

- *Nuts and seeds*: Almonds, walnuts, chia seeds and flax seeds are excellent sources of fiber and healthy fats, which help soften stools and improve bowel regularity.

▸ **Water**: Staying hydrated is essential for proper bowel function. Drinking enough water helps soften stool and facilitates its passage through the digestive tract. It is recommended that you drink 8 to 10 glasses of water daily.

▸ **Hot beverages**: Warm beverages, such as caffeine-free herbal teas, help stimulate the digestive system and promote bowel movement. Some beneficial options include chamomile tea, peppermint tea and ginger tea.

▸ **Olive or coconut oil**: Olive and coconut oils are healthy fats that can help lubricate the digestive tract and facilitate the passage of stool. You should consume a tablespoon of coconut oil or extra-virgin olive oil on an empty stomach, or add it to salads and meals.

▸ **Probiotics**: Probiotics are beneficial microorganisms that help balance intestinal flora and improve digestive health. You can find probiotics in foods such as yogurt, kefir, sauerkraut and kimchi. You may also consider taking probiotic supplements after consulting with a health professional.

▸ **Dried fruits**: Dried fruits, such as prunes and dried apricots, are fiber-rich and help relieve constipation. Add them to your cereal or yogurt, or enjoy them as a healthy snack.

▸ **Plum juice**: Plum juice is known for its natural laxative effect and can relieve occasional constipation. However, it is essential to consume it in moderation, as too much can cause diarrhea.

Remember, it's important to gradually incorporate these foods and beverages into your diet and observe how your body responds.

## Foods and Beverages to Limit or Avoid

Constipation is a common digestive issue that affects people of all ages and at various stages of life. While adopting healthy eating habits and increasing fiber intake are key steps to alleviating this problem, it is equally essential to identify the foods and beverages that may worsen the condition.

Below, you'll find a detailed list of foods and beverages to limit or avoid if you suffer from constipation, helping your digestive system work more efficiently.

▸ **Low-fiber foods**: Consuming low-fiber foods can exacerbate constipation because they lack the necessary bulk and softness to form a stool. Low-fiber foods include processed and refined foods, such as bakery products made with white flour, convenience foods, processed snack foods, and canned foods.

▸ **Dairy and dairy products**: Some people may experience constipation due to lactose intolerance. Dairy products, such as milk, cheese and yogurt, can cause constipation in these people. If you suspect you are lactose intolerant, it is advisable to limit or avoid dairy consumption and try lactose-free alternatives, such as almond milk or soy milk.

▸ **Red meat and fatty foods**: Red meat and fatty foods, such as beef and pork, as well as fried foods, can be challenging to digest and slow intestinal transit. They can contribute to constipation, so it is advisable to reduce their consumption. Instead, opt for lean protein sources, such as chicken, turkey, fish and legumes.

▸ **Processed and high-sugar foods**: Consuming processed and high-sugar foods, such as sweets, soft drinks, sugary cereals, and cookies, can exacerbate constipation. These foods are often low in fiber and high in saturated fats and refined sugars, which can affect digestion and bowel transit. Opt for more natural and healthy foods, such as fresh fruits, vegetables and whole grains.

▸ **Caffeinated beverages**: Caffeinated beverages, such as coffee and black tea, can cause dehydration and affect bowel function. If you are prone to constipation, it is advisable to limit or avoid their consumption and opt for non-caffeinated options, such as herbal tea or water.

▸ **Green bananas**: Although they are an excellent source of potassium and fiber, they can worsen constipation. This is because they contain high levels of resistant starch, which is harder to digest. Opt for ripe bananas to help relieve constipation.

▸ **Alcoholic beverages**: Excessive alcohol consumption can dehydrate the body and affect bowel function. This can lead to constipation. Limit your alcohol consumption and stay well-hydrated with water or other healthy beverages.

▸ **Carbonated beverages**: Carbonated beverages, such as soft drinks and soda, can cause bloating and abdominal discomfort and worsen constipation in some people. They generally lack nutrients and can be replaced with healthier options, such as water.

▸ **Foods that cause gas**: Certain foods, such as legumes like beans, lentils, and chickpeas, as well as specific vegetables and fruits like broccoli, cauliflower, Brussels sprouts, and apples, may be more likely to cause gas and bloating, which can exacerbate constipation. If you experience gas and constipation, it is advisable to limit your intake of these foods or look for cooking methods that make them easier to digest, such as soaking legumes before cooking or steaming vegetables.

Keep in mind that everyone responds differently to foods and beverages. If you suspect certain foods might be aggravating your constipation, it's recommended to maintain a detailed record of your diet and symptoms to identify potential triggers.

# Constipation Support: Easy and Tasty Recipes

Here is a variety of quick, easy, tasty, and healthy recipes for constipation:

## Breakfast Options

**1. Oatmeal with chia seeds and fruit**: To increase fiber, prepare a bowl of cooked oatmeal and add chia seeds. Then, add fiber-rich fruits such as bananas, strawberries, or blueberries. If you wish, you can sweeten it with honey or maple syrup.

**2. Yogurt with granola and nuts**: Choose plain, unsweetened yogurt and mix it with homemade or store-bought granola without added sugar. Add a handful of nuts, such as almonds, walnuts, or Brazil nuts, which are rich in fiber.

**3. Spinach and fruit smoothie**: Blend fresh spinach, banana, pineapple, or mango with water or vegetable milk. This smoothie is rich in fiber and nutrients that can help with intestinal transit.

**4. Whole wheat bread with avocado and egg**: Toast a slice of bread and spread it with mashed avocado. Place a poached or scrambled egg on top. This fiber, healthy fats, and protein combination can help regulate intestinal transit.

**5. Kiwi and spinach smoothie**: Blend peeled kiwi, fresh spinach, a little Greek yogurt, and water in a blender. To increase fiber, add a tablespoon of flax or chia seeds.

**6. Rye toast with mashed black beans**: Spread mashed black beans on rye toast. Black beans are rich in fiber and protein, which helps promote healthy digestion.

**7. Oatmeal-banana pancakes**: Blend oatmeal, ripe banana, eggs and a little milk until smooth. Cook the pancakes in a non-stick pan and serve them with fresh fruit and a drizzle of honey or maple syrup.

**8. Egg white omelet with spinach**: Beat egg whites with chopped spinach and season to taste. Cook the omelet in a non-stick skillet until firm. Serve with a slice of toasted whole wheat bread.

**9. Plum and wheat bran smoothie**: Blend dried plums, plain yogurt, wheat bran and a little water until smooth. Wheat bran is high in fiber and can help relieve constipation.

**10. Avocado and egg toast**: Toast a slice of whole wheat bread and spread it with mashed avocado. Cook a poached or scrambled egg and place it on the avocado. Add salt, pepper, and a touch of lemon for more flavor.

**11. Papaya and ginger smoothie**: Blend ripe papaya, cut into chunks, with grated fresh ginger and water. Papaya is known for its digestive properties; ginger can help relieve constipation.

## Lunch Creations

**1. Spinach and lentil salad**: Combine fresh spinach, cooked lentils, cherry tomatoes, cucumber and avocado in a bowl. Dress with olive oil, lemon juice and salt. Spinach and lentils are rich in fiber.

**2. Grilled chicken with steamed vegetables**: Grill a chicken fillet and serve it with steamed vegetables, such as broccoli, carrots and cauliflower. Vegetables provide fiber and help promote bowel movements.

**3. Vegetable soup**: Prepare a homemade soup with low-sodium broth and various vegetables such as carrots, zucchini, celery and spinach. Add a pinch of cumin or ginger to improve digestion.

**4. Baked fish with quinoa**: Bake a fish fillet such as salmon or hake, and serve it with cooked quinoa. Quinoa is a rich source of fiber, and the fish is rich in omega-3 fatty acids, which can also help alleviate constipation.

**5. Black bean tacos**: Prepare delicious tacos using corn or whole wheat tortillas. Fill them with cooked black beans and condiments such as cilantro, chopped onion and homemade tomato sauce. Black beans are rich in fiber and promote bowel regularity.

**6. Quinoa and vegetable salad**: Cook quinoa and let it cool. Then, mix quinoa with fresh vegetables such as cucumber, tomato, bell pepper, and onion. Add a light dressing of lemon and olive oil. Quinoa and vegetables are rich in fiber, which helps maintain a healthy digestive system.

**7. Fruit and flaxseed smoothie**: Blend fiber-rich fruits such as bananas, peaches and berries with a tablespoon of ground flaxseed. Add a little water or vegetable milk to obtain the desired consistency. Fruit smoothies are a great way to increase fiber intake and stay hydrated.

**8. Whole wheat pasta with vegetables**: Cook whole wheat pasta and combine it with sautéed vegetables such as broccoli, mushrooms, spinach and peppers. Add a little olive oil and seasonings of your choice. Whole wheat pasta contains more fiber than regular pasta, which can be beneficial for alleviating constipation.

**9. Chicken and avocado wraps**: Wrap whole wheat tortillas with grilled chicken, sliced avocado, lettuce and tomato. Add a low-fat dressing. Whole wheat wraps and avocado are rich in fiber and promote bowel regularity.

**10. Lentil soup**: Cook lentils in vegetable broth with carrots, celery and onion. Season with spices such as cumin and paprika. Lentils are an excellent source of fiber, helping to maintain a healthy digestive system.

**11. Chickpea salad**: Mix cooked chickpeas with cucumber, tomato, red onion and fresh parsley. Dress with olive oil, lemon juice, salt and pepper. Chickpeas are rich in fiber and help promote regular bowel movements.

**12. Avocado and egg toast**: Toast whole wheat bread and spread with ripe avocado. Add a boiled or scrambled egg on top. Avocados and whole wheat bread are sources of fiber, while eggs provide protein.

**13. Brown rice with steamed vegetables**: Cook brown rice and serve it with steamed vegetables such as asparagus, cauliflower, carrots and broccoli. Add a little olive oil and spices for flavor. Brown rice is rich in fiber, and the vegetables provide essential nutrients for maintaining digestive health.

**14. Pineapple and ginger smoothie**: Blend fresh pineapple, spinach, grated ginger, and water until smooth. Ginger has digestive properties, and pineapple is a fiber-rich fruit that can help relieve constipation.

**15. Chia pudding**: Mix vegetable milk, chia seeds, and a natural sweetener such as honey or maple syrup. Refrigerate the pudding for at least 2 hours or overnight to allow the chia seeds to absorb the liquid and form a gelatinous texture. For added flavor and texture, consider adding fresh fruit or nuts. Chia seeds are an excellent source of fiber, helping to regulate intestinal transit.

**16. Vegetable Frittata**: Prepare a frittata using egg whites and various vegetables, such as spinach, mushrooms, tomatoes and onions. Cook in a skillet until firm and golden brown. Egg whites are low in fat and rich in protein, while vegetables provide fiber and essential nutrients.

Remember that dietary fiber should be consumed with sufficient fluids to be effective in relieving constipation. Additionally, it is essential to consider individual nutritional needs and restrictions.

## Snacks

**1. Apple with almond butter**: Slice an apple and spread it with almond butter, which is rich in fiber and healthy fats. Sprinkle a little cinnamon for extra flavor.

**2. Carrot sticks with hummus**: Cut carrots into sticks and serve with homemade or store-bought hummus. Carrots are high in fiber, and hummus provides protein and healthy fats.

**3. Oatmeal raisin cookies**: Prepare homemade cookies with oatmeal, raisins, and a little honey as the sweetener. These cookies are high in fiber and can be a healthy option for a satisfying snack.

**4. Cucumber and salmon rolls**: Cut cucumber strips and place a slice of smoked salmon on top. Roll the two ingredients together and secure with a toothpick. This snack is low in calories and rich in fiber and omega-3 fatty acids.

**5. Yogurt with flaxseed and fruit**: Mix plain unsweetened yogurt with a tablespoon of flaxseeds and add fresh fruit, such as a pear, an apple, or berries. Flaxseeds are an excellent source of fiber and omega-3 fatty acids.

**6. Oatmeal and nut bars**: Prepare homemade bars with oatmeal, chopped nuts (such as walnuts, almonds, or pistachios), dates, and a little honey or maple syrup to sweeten. These bars are rich in fiber and nutrients.

**7. Chia pudding with fruit**: Mix vegetable milk with chia seeds and sweeten with honey or maple syrup. Let stand for at least 30 minutes so the chia seeds absorb the liquid and form a pudding. Add fresh fruit on top.

**8. Ham and asparagus rolls**: Wrap cooked asparagus in slices of low-fat ham. This snack is low in calories and rich in fiber and protein.

**9. Carrot and Walnut Muffins**: Prepare homemade muffins with whole wheat flour, grated carrots, chopped walnuts, and a little honey as a sweetener. These muffins are rich in fiber and nutrients.

**10. Celery sticks with peanut butter**: Cut celery into sticks and spread them with natural peanut butter. Celery is high in fiber, and peanut butter provides protein and healthy fats.

**11. Spinach and pineapple green smoothie**: Blend fresh spinach, pineapple chunks, a little Greek yogurt, and water in a blender. Combining fiber from spinach and pineapple can help promote healthy digestion.

Remember that a balanced diet, drinking enough water, and leading an active lifestyle are essential for promoting good intestinal health.

## Dinner Ideas

**1. Beet and Orange Salad**: Toss grated beets, orange slices, fresh spinach and walnuts in a bowl. Dress with a light lemon and olive oil vinaigrette. Beets are rich in fiber, and oranges contain vitamin C and fiber, which help promote bowel regularity.

**2. Pumpkin soup**: Prepare a roasted soup with vegetable broth, diced pumpkin, onion, garlic, and spices such as rosemary or nutmeg. Blend until smooth. Pumpkin is high in fiber and helps maintain a healthy digestive system.

**3. Spinach quiche**: Prepare a whole wheat dough base and fill it with spinach, egg whites, low-fat cheese and spices. Bake until firm and golden brown. Spinach is rich in fiber, and eggs provide protein.

**4. Fruit salad with yogurt and granola**: Combine fresh fruits such as apples, pears, strawberries and pineapple in a bowl. Add plain unsweetened yogurt and sprinkle some granola on top. The fruits are a good source of fiber, and the yogurt contains probiotics that promote gut health.

**5. Bean and vegetable burritos**: Fill whole wheat tortillas with cooked black beans, peppers, onion, corn and sautéed spinach. For an extra flavor boost, add a dash of hot sauce or a dollop of guacamole. Beans and vegetables are high in fiber and promote bowel regularity.

**6. Vegetable Gazpacho**: Prepare a refreshing gazpacho with tomatoes, cucumber, bell pepper, onion and garlic. Blend all the ingredients with olive oil, apple cider vinegar and salt. Gazpacho is a great way to increase fiber and fluid intake.

**7. Quinoa and nuts salad**: Mix cooked quinoa with nuts such as walnuts, almonds and raisins. Add fresh greens, such as spinach or arugula, and dress with a dressing made from olive oil and balsamic vinegar. Quinoa and nuts are rich in fiber and essential nutrients.

**8. Baked chicken with mashed sweet potato**: Season a chicken fillet with spices and bake it. Serve it with mashed sweet potato. Sweet potatoes are a source of fiber, and chicken provides lean protein.

**9. Spinach and Kiwi Green Smoothie**: Blend fresh spinach, peeled kiwi, banana, plain unsweetened yogurt and a little water in a blender until smooth. This smoothie is rich in fiber and nutrients that promote digestive health.

**10. Lentil and vegetable soup**: Cook lentils with broth, carrots, celery, onion, and spices such as cumin and paprika. This soup is rich in fiber and nutrients that promote digestive health.

**11. Chickpea and spinach salad**: In a bowl, mix cooked chickpeas, baby spinach, cherry tomatoes, cucumber and olives. Dress with a lemon and olive oil vinaigrette. Chickpeas and spinach are rich in fiber, which helps promote regular bowel movements.

**12. Avocado and salmon toast**: Toast whole wheat bread and spread it with ripe avocado. Add a few slices of smoked salmon and some arugula leaves. The avocado and whole wheat bread are sources of fiber, while the salmon provides omega-3 fatty acids that help maintain a healthy digestive system.

**13. Apple-oatmeal smoothie**: Blend a diced apple, plain unsweetened yogurt, oatmeal and a little cinnamon until smooth. Apple and oatmeal are sources of fiber that help promote bowel regularity.

**14. Brown rice and roasted vegetable salad**: Combine cooked brown rice with roasted vegetables such as zucchini, eggplant, peppers and onion. Dress with a light lemon and olive oil vinaigrette. Brown rice and roasted vegetables provide fiber and essential nutrients to support healthy digestion.

**15. Papaya and flaxseed smoothie**: Blend ripe papaya chunks, plain unsweetened yogurt, almond milk, and a tablespoon of ground flaxseed until smooth. Papaya is rich in digestive enzymes, and flaxseed is an excellent source of fiber that helps regulate intestinal transit.

**16. Kale and apple salad**: Combine chopped kale leaves, diced apple, walnuts and feta cheese in a bowl. Dress with a

Dijon mustard vinaigrette and olive oil. Kale and apples are rich in fiber and nutrients that promote digestive health.

**17. Chicken and vegetable wrap**: Wrap grilled chicken breast, spinach, shredded carrots, and avocado in a whole wheat tortilla. You can add a little yogurt and mustard sauce for an extra flavor boost. This option is high in fiber and lean protein to help maintain a healthy digestive system.

**18. Oat and chia pudding**: Mix oats, chia seeds, unsweetened almond milk, and a natural sweetener such as honey or maple syrup. Let the mixture sit in the refrigerator for at least 4 hours, or overnight, for the ingredients to blend and become creamy. This recipe is rich in fiber and essential nutrients for good digestion.

**19. Quinoa and steamed vegetable salad**: Cook and serve with steamed vegetables such as broccoli, carrots, zucchini and peppers. Dress with lemon juice, olive oil and spices. Quinoa and vegetables provide fiber and nutrients that promote bowel regularity.

Remember to stay hydrated and increase your consumption of liquids, such as water and natural juices, to promote intestinal transit.

# JUICES AND SMOOTHIES

*"Optimal nutrition is the medicine of tomorrow" (Dr. Linus Pauling)*

Raw foods, often referred to as "living" foods, are an exceptional source of vitamins, minerals, fiber, trace elements, enzymes, and other vital compounds that support overall health. Incorporating these nutrient-rich foods into your daily diet not only aids in disease prevention but also alleviates symptoms of various health conditions, slows down the aging process, balances gut flora, and enhances energy levels and vitality.

While salads, whole fruits, and nuts are excellent raw food options, one of the easiest and most convenient ways to ensure regular intake is by preparing homemade juices, smoothies, and shakes. These beverages serve as a delicious and practical alternative for individuals who may not enjoy consuming fruits and vegetables directly, making it easier to include these essential nutrients in their diet.

In today's world, where ultra-processed foods and toxins have become increasingly prevalent, the need for natural, nutrient-dense foods is more crucial than ever. Raw foods play a vital role in supporting detoxification, maintaining health, and restoring balance to the body.

Many people tend to prepare their juices and smoothies using only fruits, often overlooking the incredible health benefits vegetables and leafy greens provide. Adding these to your recipes not only increases variety but also significantly boosts their nutritional value, enhancing their antioxidant, remineralizing, toning, and alkalizing properties. These qualities help maintain the body's balance, rejuvenate cells, and promote overall well-being. Additionally, vegetables and greens lower the glycemic index, improve satiety, and maximize the health benefits of these preparations.

However, it is crucial to understand that most store-bought juices are far from healthy options. These commercial products are often loaded with excessive added sugars, artificial sweeteners, preservatives, and harmful chemical additives. Furthermore, the pasteurization processes used during production strip away essential vitamins and enzymes, rendering them nutritionally deficient. The high level of refinement also removes fiber, a vital component of whole foods. In many cases, these juices contain only minimal amounts of actual fruit, making them highly processed and lacking true nutritional value.

One major concern with many juices and smoothies is their high glycemic index, which can cause blood sugar spikes, lead to weight gain, and contribute to long-term metabolic imbalances. To truly enjoy healthy and nourishing beverages, the best approach is to prepare them at home using fresh, natural, and high-quality ingredients. Homemade juices and smoothies are packed with nutrients that provide genuine benefits for your body and overall well-being.

Incorporating fresh juices made from fruits, vegetables, and leafy greens into your daily routine is an excellent practice for maintaining a healthy and energetic body. With endless combinations to explore, you can enjoy not only flavorful and refreshing options but also targeted health benefits, such as relief from conditions like arthritis, thanks to essential nutrients that support wellness. Making this a part of your everyday life can transform your health, boost your energy, and elevate your quality of life. Try it for yourself and feel the difference!

## Juices: Unleash Their Power

Including smoothies or shakes in your daily diet can be an excellent way to improve your health and overall well-being. Here are some of their key benefits:

▸ **Compliance with Recommended Fruit and Vegetable**

**Intake**: Smoothies and shakes offer a practical and enjoyable way to meet the daily recommendation of five servings of fruits and vegetables. They provide a diverse range of essential nutrients that support optimal health and overall well-being.

▸ **Easy Assimilation and Digestion**: As liquid meals, smoothies and shakes are gentler on the digestive system and allow for quicker nutrient absorption. They are especially beneficial for individuals with digestive sensitivities or challenges.

▸ **Vitamin and Mineral Powerhouse**: Made from fresh fruits and vegetables, smoothies and shakes are rich sources of essential vitamins and minerals that promote the proper functioning of the body.

▸ **Detoxification and Cleansing**: Ingredients like leafy greens and natural antioxidants help flush out toxins, enhance cell health, and support effective internal cleansing.

▸ **Balancing Body pH**: By incorporating alkaline foods, smoothies and shakes play a key role in stabilizing the body's pH levels, aiding disease prevention and improving overall wellness.

▸ **Reduction of Inflammation**: Anti-inflammatory additions such as turmeric, ginger, and leafy greens can help minimize inflammation, fostering better health and increased comfort.

▸ **A Balanced Meal Replacement**: When combined with protein, healthy fats, and complex carbohydrates, smoothies become a nourishing and balanced meal replacement. They provide sustained energy and promote fullness throughout the day.

▸ **Supports Weight Management**: With their low-calorie yet nutrient-dense profiles, smoothies and shakes encourage healthy eating habits. They help manage appetite and support maintaining or achieving an ideal weight.

‣ **Enhances Skin Health**: Packed with skin-friendly vitamins like A and C from fresh ingredients, smoothies and shakes contribute to hydrated, radiant, and healthy skin.

‣ **Slows Cellular Aging**: The antioxidants in smoothie ingredients combat oxidative damage, protect cells, and help maintain a youthful appearance.

‣ **Boosts Energy and Vitality**: Smoothies made with superfoods provide a steady energy boost, helping you stay active, energized, and revitalized throughout the day.

Smoothies and shakes are a nutritious, practical, and versatile option to incorporate into your diet. In addition to making it easier to consume fruits and vegetables daily, they offer a variety of benefits for your health and overall well-being, all in a delicious and easy-to-enjoy way.

## Homemade vs. Commercial Juices

Nowadays, identifying which foods truly benefit our health can be quite challenging. Supermarkets are overflowing with an extensive range of options, flaunting attractive packaging and clever designs that promise to be natural and healthy. While advertising and packaging often catch our attention, are we genuinely purchasing natural beverages made from fruits and vegetables? Do you know the key differences between homemade juices and industrial products? Are packaged products really as nutritious as they claim to be? Taking a few moments to carefully read ingredient labels and analyze their composition may uncover some surprising truths.

A few years ago, international regulations were established to define the standards that every fruit-based beverage must meet, specifying precise characteristics for each type of product. Below, we'll explore these distinctions and delve into the essential differences.

‣ **Fruit Juice**

Fruit juice is derived from fresh, chilled, or frozen fruits without undergoing any fermentation. It may contain separately extracted pulp and, in some cases, be blended with juice from various fruits. Labels are required to specify the composition in descending order, including the exact percentage of each fruit.

To prolong shelf life and eliminate the need for refrigeration, fruit juice is typically sterilized or pasteurized. Unfortunately, these processes result in significant nutrient loss, particularly impacting essential vitamins and enzymes. Moreover, the juice lacks the natural fiber found in whole fruits.

### ▸ Juice from Concentrates

Juice from concentrates is created by reconstituting dehydrated juice concentrates with water. Concentrates are produced by extracting natural juice through evaporation or other physical methods. During reconstitution, manufacturers may add aromas or pulp from similar fruits to partially restore flavor.

Though widely consumed, these juices suffer nutrient losses during production, including enzymes, vitamins, minerals, and the valuable fiber that characterizes natural fruit.

### ▸ Dehydrated or Powdered Fruit Juice

This product is manufactured by removing water from fruit to create a dry powder, which can later be rehydrated or sold in its dehydrated state. However, the dehydration process significantly diminishes its nutritional value, leading to the loss of enzymes, vitamins, minerals, and natural fiber.

### ▸ Fruit Nectar

Fruit nectar differs from pure juice as it is made using fruit concentrate, water, and added sugars or sweeteners. Its nutritional value is considerably lower compared to natural fruit juices due to its inclusion of artificial additives to enhance flavor, color, or shelf life.

### ▸ Juice-Based Drinks

These beverages typically combine various fruits but contain minimal actual fruit juice. Often, they lack the essential nutrients derived from fruits, consisting largely of water, artificial aromas, colorings, and sweeteners.

### ▸ Milk-Infused Juice Drinks

Milk-infused juice drinks include fruit juice, often from concentrates, in very small proportions. They are mixed with milk, water, flavorings, and other ingredients. These beverages are not considered true juices, and any nutrients present are artificially added during manufacturing to compensate for losses incurred during processing.

### ▸ Vegetable and/or Greens Juice

Vegetable and greens juices are extracted from vegetables using specialized industrial methods, often with added pulp or pureed ingredients. They may also blend various vegetables to create balanced or palatable flavors.

To extend shelf life and eliminate refrigeration requirements, these juices undergo pasteurization or sterilization, which unfortunately reduces essential nutrients, including vitamins and phytonutrients. Additionally, they lack the natural fiber of whole vegetables and may include preservatives, salt, or flavor enhancers that compromise their nutritional profile.

### ▸ Commercial Smoothies

Commercial smoothies are typically prepared by blending fruits, vegetables, and greens–often using purees or concentrates–with water, milk, plant-based beverages, or similar liquids. Their thicker texture comes from a higher proportion of pulp or fiber-rich components.

To enhance taste, appearance, and shelf life, industrial smoothies usually contain added sugars, preservatives, colorings, and flavorings that alter their natural composition. Moreover, they undergo pasteurization or thermal sterilization to allow room-temperature storage, further degrading their original nutrients and reducing their overall nutritional quality.

## Advantages of Homemade Juices

After discovering what commercial products truly contain, it becomes evident that making juices at home offers numerous advantages. Here are the key benefits:

▸ **Complete Control Over Ingredients**: Preparing your own juices allows you to ensure the quality of the ingredients you use. There are no unnecessary additives, no preservatives, and–most importantly–no unpleasant surprises.

‣ **Variety and Creativity**: You have the freedom to choose your favorite fruits and vegetables, experiment with unique combinations, or incorporate fresh, seasonal produce. This not only provides a burst of delicious flavors but also boosts your intake of essential nutrients.

‣ **Authentic Aroma and Flavor**: Homemade juices retain the genuine aroma and taste of fresh fruits and vegetables. There's truly nothing like enjoying a freshly made juice packed with natural freshness.

‣ **Maximum Nutrient Retention**: Vitamins, minerals, enzymes, antioxidants, and other nutrients remain intact when you prepare juices at home, significantly enhancing their health benefits.

‣ **Premium Quality Ingredients**: Choosing fresh, seasonal produce at its peak ripeness ensures optimal flavor and exceptional nutritional value.

‣ **Seasonal Food Benefits**: Consuming fruits and vegetables that are in season supports sustainability, is more cost-effective, and often results in better taste and nutritional quality.

‣ **Total Customization**: Whether using a juicer or blender, you can adjust the consistency of your juice to your liking– whether you prefer a light, clear juice or a thicker, fiber-rich option.

‣ **Kid-Friendly Option**: Homemade juices are an excellent way to incorporate fruits and vegetables into children's diets, especially for picky eaters. With creative flavors and fun presentations, you can make juices irresistible for kids.

Making juices at home provides several compelling advantages: complete control over ingredients, enhanced nutrient retention, and the flexibility to tailor your drinks to your preferences. It's also a simple yet effective way to promote healthy eating for the whole family.

## Possible Adverse Effects

If you suffer from **gastritis, colitis, SIBO, irritable bowel syndrome, or constipation**, it's essential to take certain precautions when preparing smoothies or juices. Following these recommendations will help you enjoy their benefits without worsening your symptoms:

▸ **Use a juicer instead of a blender**: For digestive health conditions, it's often better to use a juicer rather than a blender when making juices. Juicing removes most of the fiber from the ingredients, resulting in a smoother liquid that is gentler on your digestive system.

▸ **Moderate your fiber intake**: Although fiber is highly beneficial for overall health, excessive consumption can lead to gas, bloating, or constipation–especially for individuals with sensitive digestion. Be mindful of the fiber content in your smoothies by limiting ingredients like fruit pulp, seeds, and whole grains.

▸ **Introduce juices gradually**: If you're unsure how your body will react, start with small portions. This enables you to monitor their effects on your digestion and adjust the recipes to suit your specific needs.

▸ **Consume juices on an empty stomach**: Drinking juices on an empty stomach can maximize nutrient absorption and aid digestion. This approach minimizes the risk of digestive discomfort and helps you fully benefit from the juice's nutrients.

▸ **Tailor recipes to your personal needs**: Everyone's digestive system is unique, and responses to certain foods can vary greatly. Pay close attention to how your body reacts after consuming juices, and adapt ingredient combinations to best support your health and well-being.

## When to Take Them

There are several effective ways to incorporate juices into your routine, depending on your goals and daily habits. Below are three recommended methods:

▸ **In the morning, on an empty stomach**: Begin your day with a carefully chosen juice recipe, consuming it before eating anything else. Drinking juice on an empty stomach enhances nutrient absorption and stimulates your digestive system, helping prepare it for the rest of the day.

▸ **On an empty stomach, before meals**: Enjoy a juice approximately 30 minutes before your main meals to maximize its benefits. This practice supports digestion and boosts nutrient absorption, promoting overall health and well-being.

▸ **Juice-based fasting**: Engage in a multi-day fast consisting exclusively of juices to achieve specific health objectives or to detoxify your body. Choose 2 to 3 recipes and consume them consistently throughout the day to stay nourished and energized.

## Preparation Tips

Preparing fresh juices is an easy and nutritious way to make the most of the vitamins and minerals found in fruits and vegetables. To optimize the process and ensure safety, consider the following recommendations:

▸ **Choose organic ingredients**: Whenever possible, opt for organic fruits and vegetables. They provide cleaner, pesticide-free consumption and promote a healthier lifestyle.

▸ **Wash ingredients thoroughly**: Rinse all produce carefully to remove dirt, bacteria, and chemical residues. Trim any bruised, moldy, or damaged areas to prevent contamination.

▸ **Cut ingredients into smaller pieces**: Make blending easier by chopping fruits and vegetables into smaller, manageable chunks. This helps achieve a smoother texture and shortens preparation time.

▸ **Balance ingredients with low water content**: Fruits and vegetables with low water content, such as bananas and avocados, may require pre-mixing. Start with juicier ingredients to create a liquid base, then gradually add denser items for a cohesive blend.

‣ **Peel certain fruits appropriately**: Remove citrus rinds (like those from oranges and grapefruits), as their outer layers may contain toxins. However, keep the nutrient-rich white inner layer. Peel tropical fruits, such as papayas and kiwis, especially if they are grown in regions with less stringent chemical regulations.

‣ **Discard harmful seeds**: Remove seeds from apples, as they contain trace amounts of cyanide and are unsafe to consume. On the other hand, seeds from grapes, melons, lemons, and limes are safe and offer additional health benefits.

‣ **Incorporate stems and leaves mindfully**: Many stems and leaves are nutritious, but be cautious. Avoid toxic ones, such as carrot and rhubarb leaves, which can be harmful.

‣ **Drink your juice immediately**: Freshly prepared juice is best consumed right away to minimize nutrient loss and avoid oxidation. This ensures maximum freshness and health benefits.

‣ **Remove bitter celery leaves**: Bitter celery leaves can affect the flavor of your juice. Remove them before blending the stalks to create a more balanced and enjoyable taste.

## Key Recommendations

Smoothies and shakes are an excellent, healthy alternative, but to get the most out of them, it's essential to keep certain aspects in mind. Below are some key recommendations:

‣ **Moderate fruit consumption**: Fruits are a fantastic source of nutrients but also contain fructose, a natural sugar that, when consumed excessively, can impact your health. Strive for balance by moderating your fruit intake throughout the day. Additionally, avoid eating fruits at night, as the body may metabolize them less efficiently during this time.

▸ **Choose seasonal fruits**: Seasonal fruits are often more nutrient-rich, flavorful, and cost-effective. By opting for fruits in season, you can enjoy their peak freshness and nutritional benefits while saving money.

▸ **Pick compatible combinations**: Not all fruits or ingredients blend well together. Research suitable pairings to create a smoothie or shake with balanced flavors and optimal nutritional value.

▸ **Use a moderate amount of ingredients**: The simplest smoothies are often the best. Avoid overloading them with excessive ingredients, which can lead to heavy textures or digestive discomfort. Stick to recommended recipes and be mindful of proportions.

▸ **Include leafy greens and vegetables**: Incorporate leafy greens, like spinach or kale, or vegetables, such as cucumber, to lower the glycemic index and boost your drink's nutrient profile. These additions make your smoothie both healthier and more satisfying.

▸ **Use natural sweeteners in moderation**: Enjoy the natural flavors of the ingredients, but if sweetening is necessary, choose options like raw honey or pure stevia. Use them sparingly to maintain a balanced nutritional profile.

▸ **Chew your drink**: Even liquid smoothies benefit from being "chewed." This simple habit stimulates the release of digestive enzymes, helping improve nutrient absorption and reducing discomfort like bloating or indigestion.

▸ **Store properly**: For the best results, consume smoothies or shakes fresh. If storing is needed, place them in a dark, airtight container in the refrigerator, or freeze individual portions for later use.

▸ **Make them fun and personalized**: Add an enjoyable twist by freezing smoothies in molds with fun shapes—an excellent way to turn a healthy drink into a delightful treat, especially for children.

These recommendations will help you make the most of your smoothies and shakes. While the recipes provided in this book are crafted to facilitate nutrient absorption, always remember that individual needs vary. Feel free to experiment with different combinations, tailor recipes to suit your tastes, and prioritize your health and well-being. Enjoy the journey to a healthier lifestyle!

## Nutritious Juice Recipes for Constipation

Here are some juice recipes suitable for constipation:

▸ **Prune, pear, and apple juice**
Ingredients: 4 prunes soaked overnight, 2 unpeeled pears, and 1 medium-cooked unpeeled apple. Blend the prunes with 2 tablespoons of water first. Separately blend the apples and pears. Then combine both juices and stir well.

▸ **Potato, carrot, apple and parsley juice**
Ingredients: 1 slice of potato, 4 carrots, 1 apple, and a handful of parsley. Cut the potato into strips. Cut the carrots into pieces 5 to 7 centimeters long. Cut the apple into thin slices. Blend all the ingredients.

▸ **Banana, spinach, and oat juice**
Ingredients: 1 banana, a handful of spinach, a tablespoon of oat bran, half a natural low-fat yogurt without sugar, a tablespoon of honey, and half a glass of hot water. Whisk all ingredients together and drink immediately.

▸ **Potato juice** with a teaspoon of olive oil and a little diluted sea salt. Drink a large glass.

▸ **Apple and pear juice**
Ingredients: Two or three apples and one pear. Slice the apples and the pear. Blend them, starting and ending with a few apple slices. This will be very good for you if taken before going

to sleep.

### ‣ Juice of oranges, pears and flax seeds

Ingredients: 3 oranges, 2 pears and 1½ tablespoons flax seeds. Wash the pears, remove the seeds, chop them, and place them in the blender along with the juice from the oranges and the flax seeds. Process everything until a well-blended mixture is obtained.

### ‣ Plum juice, lemon, flaxseed and ginger

Ingredients: 2 prunes, 1 lemon, 1 tablespoon of flaxseed, ½ tablespoon of ginger, and a little water. Extract the lemon juice, grate the ginger, and boil it with the prunes for 5 minutes over low heat. Then add the lemon juice and let it cool.

### ‣ Beet juice, carrots, apple and ginger

Ingredients: 1 beet, 4 carrots, ½ apples and 1½ cm ginger root slice. Blend all the ingredients.

### ‣ Cabbage or red cabbage and celery juice

Ingredients: ¼ cabbage and 3 celery stalks. Blend cabbage and celery.

### ‣ Kiwi and orange juice

Ingredients: 4 kiwis and 5 oranges. Place the peeled and chopped kiwis in the blender. Squeeze the oranges and add the juice to process everything.

### ‣ Papaya, pear and ginger juice

Ingredients: 1 papaya, 1 pear, and 1½ cm slice of ginger root. Cut the papaya and pear into pieces and add them to the blender. Blend all ingredients.

### ‣ Grape and spinach juice

The ingredients are one bunch of spinach, one bunch of grapes, and one liter of water. Blend the ingredients.

# MEDICINAL PLANTS

*"Knowledge is a treasure, but practice is its key" (Lao-Tse)*

Since time immemorial, humanity has turned to the natural world for answers to its needs. Medicinal herbs, faithful companions on this journey, have generously shared their wisdom to ease ailments and enhance well-being. This ancient knowledge, carefully preserved through the ages, has found a renewed place in the modern world, offering a healthy and sustainable option to address today's challenges.

In a society increasingly conscious of the adverse effects of certain pharmaceutical treatments and the environmental toll of unsustainable practices, botanical remedies are experiencing a resurgence with renewed prominence. For those seeking a balanced, respectful lifestyle in harmony with the environment, these green treasures provide invaluable solutions. This revival not only reflects a growing interest in ecological approaches but also an evolution toward holistic care for both the body and the planet.

What makes these natural wonders truly extraordinary is the complexity of their compounds, capable of delivering antioxidant, anti-inflammatory, antibacterial, and antiviral properties, among others. Their potential ranges from alleviating everyday issues like sleeplessness or sluggish digestion to addressing conditions such as chronic stress or age-related ailments.

Beyond the ability to target specific concerns, these species serve as vital sources of micronutrients–vitamins, minerals, fiber, and antioxidants–that fortify the immune system and support long-term health. Incorporating them into dietary or self-care routines offers a simple, sustainable, and effective path toward illness prevention and enhanced overall wellness.

The botanical kingdom boasts remarkable diversity, featuring countless species uniquely suited to meet specific needs. Whether prepared as herbal teas, applied as balms or tinctures, or utilized in the form of essential oils, their applications are as versatile as they are effective, seamlessly fitting into various lifestyles.

More than mere remedies, these natural allies inspire us to reconnect with the world around us. Harnessing their benefits requires respect for environmental rhythms and a deeper appreciation for our planet's ecosystems. Each herb or extract serves as a tangible reminder of our connection to the living world, fostering a sense of harmony that transcends the physical and nurtures the spiritual.

In addition to their myriad health benefits, plant-based solutions stand out for their accessibility and practical versatility. Many species grow abundantly in wild habitats or can be easily cultivated in home gardens, offering an affordable, sustainable alternative. In a global context marked by economic inequalities, these wellness allies provide inclusive options to complement–or even replace–costly interventions.

Over the centuries, knowledge of these natural solutions has been carefully preserved through oral traditions and written records. This heritage, rooted in deep respect for biodiversity, has been bolstered by modern science, validating the effects of their active compounds and shedding light on their mechanisms of action. It represents a powerful synergy between tradition and innovation, broadening the therapeutic applications of these botanical marvels.

However, unlocking their full potential requires responsible use. Every human body is unique, and while these species possess well-documented therapeutic properties, they are not without risks. Misuse or interactions with conventional medications can lead to adverse effects. Therefore, obtaining accurate and reliable information is essential to ensure safe and effective usage.

One particularly fascinating aspect is how the components within a plant work in unison. Whole extracts, resulting from this intricate interaction, often produce more balanced and holistic effects compared to isolated compounds. Molecules interact in complementary ways, maximizing benefits while reducing potential side effects. Conversely, isolated active principles can provide concentrated solutions but may carry an increased risk of adverse effects on the body.

The innate harmony of these botanical wonders highlights one of biodiversity's greatest gifts–balance. Whole extracts are celebrated for their gentleness and ability to integrate seamlessly with the body's natural processes. On the other hand, synthesized compounds strive for potency, often at the expense of stability. The synergistic interaction between molecular components amplifies therapeutic benefits while limiting potential downsides, making them a choice deeply aligned with human needs.

Ultimately, medicinal plants transcend their role as therapeutic tools–they bridge ancestral wisdom and scientific innovation. They remind us that the health of our bodies and the well-being of our planet are profoundly interconnected. By safeguarding this invaluable legacy, we nurture not only our own health but also that of future generations, renewing the delicate balance between humanity and nature.

## Essential Information

Although plants are natural in origin, they should not be considered entirely harmless. Their active compounds may cause adverse effects or trigger allergies in certain individuals.

Occasional consumption of an infusion is unlikely to cause harm. However, excessive, prolonged, or frequent use may result in discomfort, allergic reactions, or even toxicity.

Tolerance to natural remedies varies greatly among people. If you are pregnant, breastfeeding, or managing conditions such as chronic illnesses, allergies, kidney or liver insufficiency, cancer, or undergoing medical treatment, it is crucial to refer to the section titled **"Learn Everything You Need to Know About**

**the Plants**" before using them. This section provides essential information on potential risks, contraindications, and interactions, enabling you to make informed and responsible decisions.

## Guidelines for Care with Herbal Remedies

For best results, continue using the remedies until your symptoms have completely disappeared. The treatment duration will vary depending on factors like the severity of your condition, how it progresses, your personal commitment, and other important influences.

Keep in mind that some plants or herbal remedies are not suited for continuous or long-term use. In such cases, you will always find specific instructions that address this.

While following the guidelines for the remedies below, it is just as important to focus on the underlying causes of your symptoms. To better understand the root of your health concerns, I recommend referring to the first chapter of this book, specifically the section titled "Causes," where you'll discover essential insights into tackling the problem at its source.

Finally, remember that patience is vital. A condition that has lingered for months or years cannot be resolved in just a few days. Stay committed, persevere, and always prioritize your health and well-being.

## Measurements

To achieve the best results when preparing infusions, decoctions, or other plant-based recipes, it is essential to follow these dosage guidelines:

- A tablespoon refers to a level tablespoon.
- A teaspoon refers to a level teaspoon.

## Medicinal Plants for Constipation

In this book, we will focus on the most effective plants for eliminating or reducing constipation symptoms. The plants are detailed below, along with their various preparation methods and recommended doses. Their scientific names are indicated in parentheses, as different common names may be known in other regions and countries.

## Boldo (Peumus boldus)

*Ingredients*: 2 teaspoons of dried boldo leaves, 1 liter of water.

*Preparation*: Heat a saucepan of water. Before boiling, add the boldo and cook for 3 minutes. Remove from heat, cover, and let stand for another 2 minutes. Strain the infusion and drink it. Take 1 cup 2 or 3 times a day. Do not take Boldo for more than 4 weeks in a row.

## Cascara Sagrada (Rhamnus purshiana)

Cascara sagrada is an effective remedy for treating chronic constipation. It induces peristaltic movements and can restore regular bowel action in prolonged cases.

*Ingredients*: 1 tablespoon of dried and crushed cascara sagrada, 1 tablespoon of green anise or fennel, 300 ml of water.

*Preparation*: Boil the cascara peel with green anise or fennel for 5 minutes. Let it steep, and then drink 1 cup before going to bed. Cascara sagrada is extremely laxative, so it should not be abused. When possible, use it in a fluid extract. Also, use it with caution and do not take it for more than 2 weeks at a time, as it can cause bowel dependency.

## Chicory (Cichorium intybus)

*Ingredients*: 1 teaspoon of chicory, 300 ml of water.

*Preparation*: Boil water, then remove it from the heat. Add the chicory, cover it, and let it stand for 10 minutes. Strain the infusion and drink it before going to bed.

## Dandelion (Taraxacum officinale)

*Ingredients*: 1-2 teaspoons of dandelion, 1 glass of water.

*Preparation*: Boil the water with the dandelion for 1 minute. Remove from heat, cover, and let stand for 10 minutes. Drink this infusion 2 times a day, once in the morning and once in the afternoon.

*Cooking the root*: Ingredients: 100 grams of dandelion root and 1 liter of water.

*Preparation*: Boil the roots in water for 10 minutes. Filter the mixture and drink 3 cups daily (breakfast, lunch and dinner) for 1 month.

## Fennel (Foeniculum vulgare)

Fennel is also helpful in cases of childhood constipation.

*Ingredients*: 1 tablespoon of fennel seeds and 1 glass of water.

*Preparation*: Boil water, add fennel seeds, and remove them from the heat. Cover and let stand for 10 minutes. Strain the infusion and drink 1 cup a day.

## Frangula (Rhamnus frangula)

Frangula is effective in chronic constipation.

*Ingredients*: 1 teaspoon of frangula, 1 cup of water.

*Preparation*: Boil the water, remove it from the heat, and add the frangula. Cover and let it steep for 10 minutes. This infusion usually takes effect between 6 and 12 hours after consumption, so it is recommended to take it at night to notice its impact in the morning.

*Note*: Frangula treatments should not exceed two weeks in duration, as prolonged use may lead to dependence. Otherwise, constipation may worsen rather than improve.

# Licorice (Glycyrrhiza glabra)

Helps in the functioning of the intestine.

*Ingredients*: 1 teaspoon of dried root, 1 glass of water.

*Preparation*: Boil the water, and when it starts to boil, add the licorice and let it cook for 10 minutes. Remove from heat and let it stand for 10-15 minutes. Sweeten with honey. Drink 2 to 3 cups a day.

# Mallow (Malva sylvestris)

*Ingredients*: 2 tablespoons of dried mallow flowers and/or leaves, 1 liter of water.

*Preparation*: Slowly boil this plant's dried flowers and leaves for 15 minutes. Then, remove them from the heat and let them stand for another 10 minutes. Strain and drink. It is recommended that you drink 2 to 3 cups daily.

# Marshmallow (Althaea officinalis)

*Ingredients*: 1 teaspoon of flowers and/or dry leaves, 1 cup of water.

*Preparation*: Boil water and remove from the heat. Place the marshmallow for 10 minutes. Drink 2 cups a day.

Another way to prepare it is with *the root*. Ingredients: Add 1 or 2 tablespoons of dried root to a cup of boiling water. Let it steep overnight, strain it well, and drink 1 cup daily.

Another faster option is to use a *pulverized root*. Please follow the exact instructions as above, but ensure the water is left to stand for at least 1 hour before drinking.

# Plantain (Plantago major)

This plant is recommended for cases of chronic constipation.

*Ingredients*: 1 teaspoon of plantain seeds, 1 liter of water.

*Preparation*: Add the plantain seeds to the water and heat to boiling. Crush the seeds and let them steep for a few minutes. You can mix the infusion with honey. Drink it once or twice a day with a large amount of water.

*Another way to prepare it*: Ingredients: Put 4 or 5 chopped leaves in a liter of water and boil for 10 minutes. Please turn off the heat, let it stand for 5 minutes, strain it, and drink it. Plantain increases the volume of stool, facilitating its expulsion.

It is essential to note that drinking plenty of water is crucial for achieving results; otherwise, it may cause obstructions in the colon.

## Rhubarb (Rheum rhabarbarum)

It acts as a purgative at high doses, tones the intestinal wall at small doses, and helps fight gas.

*Ingredients*: 1 teaspoon of dried rhubarb roots, 1 glass of water.

*Preparation*: Bring the water to a boil. Remove from the heat and add the rhubarb. Let it stand for 10 minutes. Drink 1 cup before going to bed.

It should not be taken for more than 8 consecutive days.

*Warning*: Rhubarb has many contraindications. Refer to it in the section "Learn all about recommended plants."

## Senna (Cassia angustifolia)

It is a more potent laxative than frangula.

*Ingredients*: 1 tablespoon of senna leaves, 1 tablespoon of anise or fennel seeds, 1 liter of water.

*Preparation*: Boil the water. Please remove it from the heat and add the senna, anise, or fennel. Cover and let stand for 10 minutes. Strain and drink, preferably on an empty stomach. The rest should be consumed after meals.

*Another way of preparation*: Ingredients: 5 to 7 leaves or fruits and 1 glass of water. Place it in a saucepan and bring to a boil for 5 minutes. Please remove it from the fire and let it stand for another 5 minutes. Because it can cause cramps, use it only in infusion, without boiling.

Take this plant for a maximum of 8 consecutive days, as it can cause intestinal dependence.

## Herbal Remedy Recipes

Although the plants mentioned above are effective when used individually, their properties can be further enhanced when combined properly. Below are some particularly effective combinations.

### ‣ Herbal Remedy Recipe No. 1

*Ingredients*: 1/2 tablespoon of barberry, 1/2 tablespoon of boldo or dandelion, 1/2 teaspoon of cascara sagrada, 1/2 teaspoon of licorice, 1/2 teaspoon of rhubarb root, ginger or fennel (1/2 teaspoon), 300 ml of water.

*Preparation*: Drink 1 cup of this infusion before bedtime.

### ‣ Herbal Remedy Recipe No. 2

*Ingredients*: 1 tablespoon of senna leaves, 1 tablespoon of fennel seeds, 1 tablespoon of camomile flowers.

*Preparation*: Boil water, then remove it from the heat and add the senna, fennel, and chamomile. Cover and let stand for 10 minutes. (Warning: Prolonged use of this remedy is not recommended, as senna leaves can cause intestinal colic.)

### ‣ Herbal Remedy Recipe No. 3

*Ingredients*: 2 tablespoons of rhubarb in pieces, 1 tablespoon of dried senna leaves, 1 branch of mint or peppermint, 1 tablespoon of baking soda, 1 liter of water.

*Preparation*: Boil water, then remove it from the heat and add rhubarb, senna, and mint. Cover and let stand for 10-15 minutes. Strain and then add the baking soda. Drink half on an empty stomach in the morning and the other half before bed at night.

## Simple Steps to Make a Tincture for Constipation

Tinctures, also known as concentrated botanical extracts, are an effective and potent way to harness the therapeutic benefits of medicinal plants. Through a careful extraction process, essential compounds, such as phytochemicals and active principles, are obtained, providing valuable healing properties.

These liquid solutions have been used for centuries in traditional medicine due to their proven efficacy and exceptional versatility. In recent years, they have regained their relevance thanks to the growing interest in natural remedies and herbal practices.

The method for preparing these extracts can vary, but it generally involves immersing plant parts–such as roots, leaves, flowers, or bark–in a solvent like alcohol, glycerin, or water. During the steeping process, the plant's active elements are extracted into the liquid, creating a medicinal concentrate that retains its essential properties.

One of the main advantages of these preparations is their practicality. They can be administered orally by adding a few drops to water or juice, allowing for rapid absorption. Additionally, their high concentration enables precise dosage adjustments based on individual needs.

▸ **Making a Cascara Sagrada Tincture:**
*Ingredients*: 500 grams of chopped cascara sagrada, 4 liters of distilled water, and 250 ml of glycerin.

*Preparation*: Place 500 grams of chopped cascara sagrada in 4 liters of distilled water and boil vigorously until the water reduces to just covering the rind. Strain the liquid and set it aside. Return the rind to the pot, add 2 liters of water, and boil again until the water barely covers the rind. Strain and combine both liquids, then simmer over low heat until reduced to one quart, ideally using a double boiler for the final reduction to avoid burning. Add 250 ml of glycerin, mix well, let it cool, and bottle.

*Dosage*: Take ½ to 1 teaspoon of the tincture at night before bedtime. It's important not to modify or mask its natural bitterness, as much of its therapeutic efficacy derives from this characteristic.

*Storage*: Store the tincture in a cool, dark place to maintain its potency. Ensure you use it within 1 year to guarantee maximum efficacy.

## Learn Everything You Need to Know About the Plants

In this section, we'll delve into the most recommended botanical species for treating the condition at hand. You'll find essential information about their possible adverse effects, contraindications, and interactions, as well as detailed insights into each plant. From their descriptions and habitats to their uses, chemical components, histories, and therapeutic properties, this chapter is designed to take you on a fascinating journey of discovery.

My goal is to provide you with a comprehensive understanding of these plants, helping you grasp their context and fully appreciate their many benefits. We'll explore their historical origins and significance in traditional medicine, highlighting their invaluable role in natural care.

I want you to become an expert on these species, capable of making informed decisions in your pursuit of wellness. Get ready to expand your knowledge and uncover the extraordinary healing power of nature!

### Barberry (Berberis vulgaris)

**Description:**

Barberry is a deciduous shrub belonging to the Berberidaceae family. It reaches a height of approximately 1 to 3 meters and has thorny branches. The leaves are small, oval, toothed, and deep green, taking on a reddish hue in autumn. The flowers are yellow and are grouped in hanging clusters. The fruits are bright red berries.

### Habitat and cultivation:

Barberry is native to Europe but is also found in other parts of the world, such as Asia and North America. It grows in wooded areas, hedgerows, and roadsides. It prefers rich, well-drained soils and can adapt to different climatic conditions.

As for cultivation, barberry is a hardy plant that can be propagated by seed or cuttings. It is recommended to be planted in full sun or partially shaded areas. It requires regular watering and can benefit from light pruning to maintain shape and encourage healthy growth.

### Parts used:

The bark, roots and berries of barberries are used for medicinal purposes. The bark and roots are dried and used in powdered form, while the berries can be consumed fresh or dried for later use.

### Components:

Barberry contains various chemical components, including alkaloids such as berberine, oxybenzone, and palmatine. These alkaloids are responsible for many of the plant's therapeutic properties.

### History and tradition:

Barberry has been used in traditional medicine for centuries. In ancient Greece, it was considered a sacred plant for treating various conditions, including digestive disorders and skin diseases. It has also been used in traditional Chinese medicine and Indian Ayurvedic medicine.

### Therapeutic properties:

Barberry has traditionally been used for its therapeutic properties. It is attributed with antibacterial, antifungal, anti-inflammatory, and antioxidant properties. It has been used to treat gastrointestinal disorders such as diarrhea and dyspepsia, to improve liver function, and to stimulate the immune system.

In addition, the berberine in barberry has been the subject of numerous scientific studies, demonstrating its efficacy in treating various health conditions, including diabetes, cardiovascular disease, and bacterial infections.

### Curiosities:

Barberry has historically been used as a natural dye due to its ability to produce intense yellow and orange colors.

Barberry berries have a tart flavor and are used to prepare jams, jellies, and beverages, such as barberry wine.

In some cultures, barberry thorns have been used as improvised pins or needles.

Barberry is prized for its ornamental appeal due to its yellow flowers and vibrant red fruits.

Some butterfly species use barberry as a food source for their larvae.

### Adverse or side effects:

Although barberry is generally safe when used correctly, some adverse effects have been reported. These may include stomach upset, diarrhea, nausea, vomiting and skin rashes. In addition, excessive consumption of barberry or prolonged use may result in liver damage. If any adverse reactions occur, discontinue use and seek medical attention immediately.

### Contraindications:

There are some contraindications and precautions to keep in mind when using barberry:

Pregnancy and lactation: Barberry should be avoided during these periods due to a lack of sufficient information.

Gastrointestinal problems: people with gastrointestinal diseases, such as ulcers, Crohn's disease, or ulcerative colitis, should avoid barberry because it stimulates intestinal activity and may worsen symptoms.

Liver disease: Barberry may cause liver damage, so people with liver disease should avoid it.

**Interactions:**
It may interact with certain medications and supplements. Some known interactions include:

Medications that are metabolized in the liver: The berberine present in barberry may affect the liver enzymes responsible for metabolizing certain drugs, potentially altering their effectiveness or increasing side effects. Caution is advised when combining barberry with medications that are processed in the liver, such as some antidepressants, statins and anticoagulants.

Blood pressure medications: Barberry may have a hypotensive effect, so its combination with drugs for low blood pressure could potentiate this effect and cause an excessive decrease in blood pressure.

# Boldo (Peumus boldus)

**Description:**
Boldo is a perennial shrub in the Monimiaceae family. It is native to South America, specifically Chile, and has spread to other regions with similar climates. Boldo has leathery, lanceolate, dark green leaves. When ripe, its tiny yellow flowers produce small, round black fruits. Its intense aroma and bitter taste characterize Boldo.

**Habitat and cultivation:**
Boldo grows wild in mountainous areas with Mediterranean and subtropical climates. It requires well-drained soils and prefers areas with sun exposure. As for its cultivation, it can be propagated through seeds, although it is also commonly reproduced by cuttings. It is a hardy plant and can tolerate drought conditions.

**Parts used:**
The parts of boldo used are mainly the leaves. These are harvested manually and dried for later use. The dried leaves contain beneficial compounds that provide medicinal properties.

**Components:**
Boldo contains several chemical components that give it its therapeutic properties. Some of the main elements include alkaloids (such as boldine), flavonoids, essential oils, tannins, and antioxidant compounds. These compounds contribute to the medicinal properties of boldo.

**History and tradition:**
Boldo has a long history of use in traditional South American medicine. The indigenous peoples of Chile used it to treat various digestive disorders, such as indigestion and colic. In some cultures, it is also considered a sacred plant and has been used in rituals and ceremonies to purify the body and spirit.

**Therapeutic properties:**
It is used primarily for its digestive and hepatic properties. Some of the therapeutic benefits associated with Boldo include:

It stimulates bile production and aids in the digestion of fats.
It relieves digestive disorders such as indigestion, stomach upset, and gas.
It protects and stimulates liver function, helping detoxify the body.
It has antioxidant and anti-inflammatory properties.
It is traditionally used as a mild diuretic to relieve symptoms of cystitis.

**Curiosities:**
Boldo is a plant highly appreciated in traditional medicine in South America. It is also used to prepare beverages and liquors, such as the famous "pisco sour" in Chile.

In some countries, such as Argentina and Chile, boldo is considered a national symbol of healing and protective properties.

In popular tradition, boldo is said to help relieve hangovers and stomach upset caused by excessive alcohol consumption.

**Adverse or side effects:**
It is generally considered safe when consumed in moderate amounts. However, some people may experience adverse effects, such as stomach upset, nausea, vomiting, or diarrhea.

Excessive consumption may irritate the stomach and kidneys and, in extreme cases, may cause liver damage.

Some people may have an allergic reaction to boldo, so caution is advised if you have a known sensitivity to plants of the Monimiaceae family.

**Contraindications:**
It is not recommended for pregnant or lactating women, as it may have uterine stimulant effects, and there is insufficient evidence of its safety in these situations.

Those with severe liver or kidney disease should avoid taking Boldo, as it may aggravate these conditions.

People with bile duct obstruction or gallstones should avoid its consumption, as it may increase symptoms or cause complications.

**Interactions:**
Boldo may interact with some medications, such as anticoagulants or antiplatelet drugs, increasing the risk of bleeding. Caution should be exercised, and a physician should be consulted for these medications.

Due to its diuretic effect, it may potentiate the effects of diuretic drugs, which could lead to increased fluid and electrolyte loss.

If you take medications metabolized by the liver, such as certain cholesterol medications or oral contraceptives, boldo may interfere with their metabolism and decrease their effectiveness.

# Cascara Sagrada (Rhamnus purshiana)

**Description:**
Cascara sagrada is an evergreen shrub that can grow up to 6 meters high. Its branches are slender and covered with thorns. The leaves are lanceolate and shiny, dark green. However, the most outstanding part is its bark, which is used for medicinal purposes.

**Habitat and cultivation:**
It is primarily found in the mountainous regions of northwestern North America, particularly in areas such as Oregon and Washington. It prefers moist, fertile soils and typically grows in temperate and humid forests. Its cultivation has been successfully carried out in various parts of the world, including Europe, where it has adapted well to areas with similar climates.

**Parts used:**
The part of the cascara that is harvested is its bark, which comes from mature trees. The bark must be processed and dried before it can be used for medicinal purposes.

**Components:**
It contains several active components that give it its therapeutic properties. Among them are anthraquinones, such as emodin and frangulin, which are responsible for its laxative effect. It also contains tannins, which give it astringent properties.

**History and tradition:**
Cascara sagrada has been used for centuries by Native American tribes, such as the Native Americans of the Pacific Northwest. These tribes considered it a sacred plant and used it to treat digestive disorders and as a purgative. European settlers learned about its properties and began using it for medicinal purposes.

**Therapeutic properties:**

It is known for its laxative and purgative properties. The active components present in its bark stimulate intestinal movement and promote evacuation. This plant is commonly used to treat occasional constipation and to regularize intestinal transit. It has also been traditionally used to relieve indigestion and as a digestive tonic.

It is essential to note that while cascara sagrada can effectively relieve occasional constipation, prolonged use or excessive doses can lead to dependence and digestive system imbalances.

**Curiosities:**
Cascara sagrada is native to North America, especially the northwestern regions of the United States and Canada.

The plant's common name, "cascara sagrada", comes from the belief that it has sacred or spiritual medicinal properties.

Native Americans have long used cascara sagrada as a natural remedy to alleviate constipation and other digestive issues.

The bark of the cascara sagrada tree contains compounds called anthraquinones, which are responsible for its laxative properties.

**Adverse or side effects:**
If consumed in high doses or for a prolonged period, cascara sagrada can cause adverse effects such as colic, severe diarrhea and electrolyte imbalances.

Some people may experience stomach upset, nausea, or vomiting after taking cascara sagrada.

Excessive or prolonged use of cascara sagrada can lead to laxative dependence, which means that the body can become dependent on its use for regular bowel movements.

Following the dosage recommendations and staying within the recommended dose is essential.

**Contraindications:**

Cascara sagrada is contraindicated in people with inflammatory bowel conditions, such as Crohn's disease or ulcerative colitis.

It is not recommended to use it during pregnancy or lactation, as its safety in these stages has not been established.

People suffering from intestinal obstruction, appendicitis, hemorrhoids, or severe abdominal problems should avoid the use of cascara sagrada.

If you are taking medications such as anticoagulants, antiarrhythmics, diuretics, or corticosteroids, it is essential to consult a physician before using cascara sagrada due to possible drug interactions.

**Interactions:**
Due to their anticoagulant effect, they may interact with certain medications such as anticoagulants. If taken together, they may increase the risk of bleeding.

It may also interfere with the absorption of other medications, such as diuretics or blood pressure medications, reducing their effectiveness.

If you are taking other medications, it is essential to talk to your doctor or pharmacist before using cascara sagrada to avoid possible negative interactions.

# Chamomile (Matricaria chamomilla)

**Description:**
Chamomile is an annual herbaceous plant in the Asteraceae family. Its erect, branched stem can reach a height of up to 60 centimeters. The leaves are finely divided and light green. The chamomile flowers are small and daisy-shaped, with a yellow center surrounded by white petals. A distinctive apple scent is released when the flowers are rubbed between the fingers.

**Habitat and cultivation:**

Chamomile is native to Europe and commonly found in temperate climate regions. It grows best in well-drained, nutrient-rich soils and can be found in meadows, fields, roadsides and gardens. Chamomile is a hardy and adaptable plant that can grow in various conditions. It can also be quickly grown from seed or by dividing existing plants.

**Parts used:**

The dried flowers are used in the chamomile parts. These are harvested when fully open and air-dried to preserve their therapeutic properties. The dried flowers are used to prepare infusions, extracts, essential oils and cosmetic products.

**Components:**

Chamomile contains various components that contribute to its therapeutic properties. These include essential oils, such as bisabolol and azulene oxide, which have anti-inflammatory and soothing properties. It also contains flavonoids, such as apigenin, which have antioxidant and anti-inflammatory properties. Other components present in chamomile include caffeic acid, coumarins and polyphenols.

**History and tradition:**

Various cultures have used chamomile since ancient times due to its therapeutic properties. The ancient Egyptians used it in religious rituals and skin care. It was also known and used in traditional Greek and Roman medicine. In popular tradition, chamomile is associated with calming and relaxing properties and has been used to relieve stress, anxiety, and sleep disorders.

**Therapeutic properties:**

Chamomile is renowned for its therapeutic properties and is used in herbal medicine for its diverse health benefits. It is attributed to anti-inflammatory, antioxidant, antibacterial, soothing, and digestive properties. Chamomile is commonly used to relieve upset stomach, colic, indigestion and nausea. It is also used to reduce stress and anxiety, as well as promote relaxation. In addition, it has been used topically to relieve skin irritation, minor burns, and skin conditions such as dermatitis and eczema.

### Curiosities:

Chamomile is an herbaceous plant of the Asteraceae family with interesting properties. For example, its name comes from the Greek "chamaimelon", which means "apple on earth", due to its characteristic apple aroma. In addition, chamomile has been used for centuries in various cultures for its therapeutic properties and is considered one of the oldest and most widely recognized herbs in herbal medicine.

### Adverse or side effects:

Chamomile is generally considered safe and well-tolerated. However, adverse effects or side effects may occur in some cases. Some people may experience allergic reactions when they come into contact with the plant or consume chamomile products. In addition, excessive consumption of chamomile may cause stomach upset, nausea, or vomiting in some people. It is essential to be aware of these possible effects, discontinue use immediately, and consult a health professional if you experience any adverse effects.

### Contraindications:

Although generally safe, specific contraindications are associated with the use of chamomile. For example, people who are allergic to other plants in the Asteraceae family, such as ragweed or sunflowers, may be at an increased risk of developing allergic reactions to chamomile. Additionally, caution is advised for pregnant or nursing women, as there have been insufficient studies conducted to determine its safety in these stages.

### Interactions:

In general, chamomile has not been associated with significant drug interactions. However, it is always advisable to consult a healthcare professional if you are taking any medications or have pre-existing health conditions before using chamomile therapeutically. Some studies suggest that chamomile may have mild anticoagulant effects, so caution should be exercised when combining it with anticoagulant or antiplatelet medications.

# Chicory (Cichorium intybus)

**Description:**
Chicory is a perennial herbaceous plant in the Asteraceae family. Its erect and branched stem can reach a height of up to one meter. The plant's leaves are lanceolate and arranged in a basal rosette. They have a marked central nerve. Chicory flowers are light blue and grouped in inflorescences as heads.

**Habitat and cultivation:**
Chicory is native to Europe but is now distributed worldwide. It prefers to grow in nutrient-rich, well-drained soils and can adapt to different climatic conditions. It is commonly found in meadows, roadsides, and vacant lots.

**Parts used:**
It is mainly grown for its roots, which are used for various purposes. After the plant has grown, the roots are harvested in autumn. The leaves and flowers are also used, although to a lesser extent.

**Components:**
This plant contains various active compounds, including sesquiterpenes, sesquiterpene lactones, inulin, tannins, flavonoids and phenolic acids. These substances confer medicinal properties and health benefits.

**History and tradition:**
They date back to ancient times. In ancient Egypt, chicory was used as food and to treat digestive problems. In the Middle Ages, it was cultivated in monasteries and used as a medicinal plant. Additionally, during the European coffee shortage, chicory root began to be used as a substitute for coffee, particularly during the war.

**Therapeutic properties:**
Chicory has been traditionally used as a digestive tonic and hepatoprotective. It is attributed to diuretic, cholagogue, and mild laxative properties. In addition, it is used in cases of liver

and gallbladder disorders, such as jaundice and dyspepsia. The plant's inulin also gives it prebiotic properties, promoting the growth of beneficial bacteria in the intestine.

### Curiosities:

It should be noted that its roasted and ground roots have been used as a substitute for coffee in some regions. The flavor of this drink is similar to coffee but milder and with a slightly bitter touch. In addition, chicory is also used as an ingredient in some alcoholic beverages, such as Angostura bitters.

Another interesting fact about chicory is that its flowers open and close in response to sunlight. During the day, the flowers open to attract pollinators, while at night, they close to protect pollen and prevent water loss.

### Adverse or side effects:

Some people, especially those sensitive to plants in the Asteraceae family, may experience allergic reactions to chicory. These reactions may include skin rashes, itching, or difficulty breathing. Additionally, excessive consumption may have a more pronounced laxative effect, potentially leading to diarrhea.

### Contraindications:

It is recommended to avoid the consumption of chicory in pregnant or breastfeeding women since there is not enough scientific evidence on its safety in these situations. Also, people suffering from bile duct obstruction or gallstones should avoid the consumption of chicory, as it may stimulate bile production and worsen symptoms.

### Interactions:

It is important to note that chicory may interact with certain medications used to treat clotting disorders, such as anticoagulants. This is because the plant contains substances that could increase the risk of bleeding in combination with these drugs.

## Dandelion (Taraxacum officinale)

**Description:**
Dandelion, whose scientific name is Taraxacum officinale, is a perennial herbaceous plant that belongs to the Asteraceae family. It is a medium-sized plant that can grow to a height of 30-40 centimeters. It has toothed leaves that form a basal rosette at the base of the plant. Its bright yellow flowers are grouped in characteristic heads resembling tiny suns. After flowering, the flowers give way to a fluffy white seed head known as a "parachute", which is easily dispersed by the wind.

**Habitat and cultivation:**
The dandelion is native to Europe and Asia, but it is now found worldwide. It is a highly adaptable plant that can grow in various habitats, including meadows, gardens, fields and roadsides. However, it is considered an invasive plant in some places because it can spread rapidly and displace other species. Regarding cultivation, dandelion is a hardy plant that can grow in almost any well-drained soil. It can also grow in both full sun and partial shade.

**Parts used:**
Both the leaves and roots of dandelion are used medicinally. The young and tender leaves can be used in salads or cooked as vegetables. On the other hand, the roots are dried and used to make infusions, extracts and tinctures.

**Components:**
Dandelion contains various beneficial health components. The leaves contain vitamins A, C, and K, as well as minerals such as iron, calcium, and potassium. The roots contain inulin, a type of soluble fiber, as well as phenolic compounds, flavonoids, and triterpenoids, which are responsible for many of the dandelion's therapeutic properties.

**History and tradition:**
Dandelion has been used in traditional medicine for centuries. Its use dates back to ancient Greece and Rome, where it was used to treat digestive and liver problems. It has also been used in traditional Chinese and Ayurvedic medicine. In addition to its medicinal properties, dandelion also has a place in cultural tradition. For example, in some European cultures, blowing

dandelion seeds is believed to bring good luck or fulfill wishes.

**Therapeutic properties:**
Dandelion has numerous therapeutic properties that make it a valuable addition to natural medicine. It has traditionally been used to stimulate digestion, relieve bloating and constipation, and promote liver and gallbladder health. In addition, dandelion has diuretic properties, which means it can help encourage the elimination of fluids and toxins from the body. It has also been used to promote kidney health and improve kidney function. Additionally, dandelion has antioxidant and anti-inflammatory properties, making it beneficial in treating inflammatory conditions, such as arthritis. However, it is essential to note that dandelion can interact with certain medications and cause allergic reactions in some people.

**Curiosities:**
The dandelion has some exciting curiosities. One of them is its name, which comes from the French "dent de lion", which means "dandelion" in Spanish. This is due to the shape of its leaves, which resemble the teeth of a lion. Another curiosity is that all parts of the dandelion are edible and have health benefits. Every part of the plant can be used in cooking or natural medicine, from the flowers to the roots. In addition, dandelion is one of the first plants to bloom in spring; its bright yellow flowers are a sign that winter is over and the growing season is in full swing.

**Adverse or side effects:**
Although dandelion is generally safe for most people, it may cause some adverse effects in some cases. The most common side effects include stomach upset, diarrhea, and allergic reactions in sensitive people. In addition, dandelion may have a diuretic effect, which can increase urine production. This can benefit some people, but can also lead to dehydration if insufficient fluid is consumed. Additionally, excessive consumption of dandelion can interact with certain medications, such as diuretics, so it is essential to exercise caution when combining it with other treatments.

**Contraindications:**

Although dandelion is considered safe for most people, there are some contraindications to be aware of. People with known allergies to plants in the Asteraceae family, such as ragweed, chrysanthemum, or daisy, should avoid consuming dandelion, as they may have allergic reactions. In addition, people who have bile duct obstruction or gallstones should avoid dandelion consumption, as it may increase bile production and worsen these problems. If you have any specific health conditions, it is advisable to consult a health professional before using dandelion.

**Interactions:**
Dandelion may interact with certain medications, so it is essential to exercise caution when combining it with other treatments. For example, dandelion may increase the effects of diuretic medications, which can lead to increased fluid and electrolyte removal from the body. Additionally, dandelion may interact with drugs metabolized in the liver, such as blood thinners, medications used to treat diabetes, and those used to lower cholesterol levels. This can affect the effectiveness and safety of these medications. If you are taking any medications, it is advisable to consult your doctor before using dandelion or supplements containing dandelion. Your doctor can evaluate possible interactions and adjust the dosage or treatment accordingly.

# Fennel (Foeniculum vulgare)

**Description:**
Fennel is a perennial herbaceous plant in the Apiaceae family. Its erect, striated stems can reach a height of up to 2 meters. The leaves are long, finely divided, and bright green. The flowers are small and yellow, grouped in umbels. Fennel produces dry, elongated fruits that contain seeds. Both the leaves and seeds have a distinctive aroma and an anise flavor.

**Habitat and cultivation:**
Fennel is native to the Mediterranean region but is cultivated in many parts of the world because of its culinary and medicinal

value. It prefers well-drained, fertile soils and can grow in full sun or partial shade. It is drought-resistant and can tolerate cold temperatures. Fennel is quickly grown from seed and is found in gardens and commercial cultivation.

**Parts used:**
The parts of fennel used for culinary and medicinal purposes are the seeds, leaves, and stems. The seeds are the most commonly used, either whole or ground. The leaves and stems can also be fresh or dried to flavor dishes.

**Components:**
Fennel contains various beneficial health components. Its seeds are rich in essential oils, such as anethole, which give it its characteristic aroma and flavor. They also contain phenolic compounds, flavonoids and phytochemicals, which have antioxidant and anti-inflammatory properties. Fennel is also a good source of dietary fiber, vitamins (C and B6), and minerals (calcium, iron and potassium).

**History and tradition:**
Fennel has a rich history of use in traditional medicine and cooking across various cultures. Indian Ayurvedic medicine has been used to treat digestive issues, including indigestion and colic. Traditional Chinese medicine has been used to improve digestion, relieve gas, and promote breastfeeding. Additionally, fennel has been used in Mediterranean cuisine for centuries for its distinctive flavor and digestive properties.

**Therapeutic properties:**
Fennel possesses therapeutic properties that make it a valuable ingredient in natural medicine. It has been used to relieve digestive issues, including indigestion, colic, and flatulence. Due to its expectorant and antispasmodic properties, it has also been used to treat respiratory conditions, such as coughs and the common cold. Fennel has also been used to stimulate appetite, promote breastfeeding, and relieve symptoms of premenstrual syndrome. In addition, its potential to reduce inflammation, improve eye health, and promote cardiovascular health has been investigated. However, it is essential to note that fennel may cause adverse effects in some

people, such as allergies.

### Curiosities:

Fennel has some interesting curiosities associated with its history and use. In ancient Greece, fennel was revered as a sacred plant used in religious ceremonies. In addition, Greek and Roman warriors used to chew fennel seeds to increase their strength and endurance. In the Middle Ages, fennel was believed to possess magical powers and was used as a talisman to ward off the evil eye and other malevolent spells. In cooking, fennel is recognized for its use in traditional dishes, such as fennel bread and liqueur, which are widely consumed in many Mediterranean countries.

### Adverse or side effects:

Although fennel is generally considered safe for most people when consumed in moderate amounts, it may cause adverse effects in some people. Some people may experience allergies to fennel, which may manifest as skin rashes, itching, or difficulty breathing. In addition, excessive consumption of fennel may cause stomach upset, diarrhea, or a burning sensation in the stomach. In rare cases, severe allergic reactions have been reported, including swelling of the face, lips, or tongue, which may require immediate medical attention.

### Contraindications:

Although fennel is generally safe for most people, there are some contraindications. Pregnant women should avoid consuming it, as it may stimulate the uterus and cause contractions, which can be dangerous during pregnancy. Caution is also recommended for lactating women, as the effects of fennel consumption on breast milk production are unknown. People with blood clotting disorders or who are taking anticoagulants should avoid it, as it may increase the risk of bleeding.

### Interactions:

Fennel may interact with certain medications, so it is essential to exercise caution when combining it with other treatments. For example, fennel may increase the effects of anticoagulant drugs, such as warfarin, increasing the risk of bleeding.

Additionally, fennel may interact with the absorption of certain medications, including proton pump inhibitors used to treat heartburn and thyroid medications. It has also been reported that fennel may have a weak estrogenic effect, so people who take hormone therapy or have a history of hormone-related cancer should use caution and consult their physician before using fennel or fennel supplements.

# Frangula (Rhamnus frangula)

### Description:
The frangula, scientifically known as Rhamnus frangula, is a perennial shrub belonging to the Rhamnaceae family. This plant, also known as black alder or kangaroo, is native to Europe, western Asia, and parts of North America. Buttercup has a distinctive appearance, with slender branches, alternate leaves, and small, greenish flowers that develop in clusters. When mature, it produces small black berries containing seeds.

### Habitat and cultivation:
It is commonly found in wet areas, such as swamps, river margins, and humid forests. It prefers fertile, well-drained soils. As for cultivation, frangula can be propagated through seeds or cuttings. However, it is essential to note that in some regions, it may be considered an invasive species, and therefore, its cultivation may be restricted.

### Parts used:
The most commonly used parts of frangula are the bark and berries. The bark is harvested from the shrub's stems and branches. Ripe berries can also be used, although to a lesser extent. The bark and the berries contain active compounds that confer medicinal properties on the plant.

### Components:
It contains several chemical components that give it its therapeutic properties. The anthraquinones, such as frangulin and emodin, are among the most important compounds. These substances are responsible for the plant's laxative and purgative

properties. Other components include flavonoids, tannins, and essential oils in smaller quantities.

### History and tradition:

Frangula has been used in traditional European medicine for centuries. It is believed that the ancient Egyptians already knew of its laxative properties. The plant is widely used in Europe to treat constipation and other digestive disorders. It has also traditionally been used as a diuretic to relieve skin conditions. Additionally, frangula has been used to produce natural dyes due to its ability to create dark tones.

### Therapeutic properties:

Frangula is primarily known for its laxative and purgative properties. The anthraquinone compounds in its bark and berries stimulate intestinal movement and promote bowel regularity, so it is used to treat occasional constipation and promote bowel regularity.

Frangula has laxative and diuretic properties. It helps increase urine production and promotes the elimination of toxins from the body.

### Curiosities:

It is known as the "black alder" because its bark resembles that of common alders.

Although primarily used for medicinal purposes, frangula has also been used to produce natural dyes, as its bark yields dark tones.

The ancient Egyptians were aware of the laxative properties of frangula and used it for this purpose.

The frangula is a plant found mainly in Europe, Western Asia, and North America.

In traditional European medicine, frangula has been used for centuries as an herbal remedy to treat constipation and other digestive problems.

**Adverse or side effects:**
Prolonged or abusive use of frangula may cause adverse effects such as severe diarrhea, colic and electrolyte imbalances.

Some people may experience stomach upset, nausea, or vomiting after taking frangula.

Frangula may also cause irritation or tenderness in the gastrointestinal tract for some people.

It is important to note that overuse of frangula can lead to dependence on laxatives, which means that the body can become dependent on their use for regular bowel movements.

**Contraindications:**
Frangula is contraindicated in cases of intestinal obstruction, appendicitis, hemorrhoids, or any severe abdominal condition.

It is not recommended to use it during pregnancy or lactation, as its safety in these stages has not been established.

Those suffering from inflammatory bowel diseases, such as Crohn's disease or ulcerative colitis, should avoid using frangula.

If you are taking medications such as anticoagulants, diuretics, antiarrhythmics, or corticosteroids, it is essential to consult a physician before using frangula due to possible drug interactions.

**Interactions:**
Frangula may interact with certain medications, such as anticoagulants, due to its anticoagulant effect. It may increase the risk of bleeding if taken together with these medications.

It may also interfere with the absorption of other medications, such as diuretics or blood pressure medications, reducing their effectiveness.

If you are taking other medications, it is essential to talk to your doctor or pharmacist before using frangula to avoid possible negative interactions.

# Ginger (Zingiber officinale)

**Description:**
Ginger is a perennial plant with underground stems called rhizomes. It has long, narrow leaves and yellow or white cone-shaped flowers. The rhizome is the most commonly used part and has a spicy and aromatic flavor.

**Habitat and cultivation:**
Ginger is native to tropical Asia and is grown in many parts of the world. It prefers warm, humid climates and can be grown both in gardens and in pots indoors.

**Parts used:**
The rhizome of ginger is the most commonly used part of the ginger plant. It is harvested, peeled, and used fresh or dried for culinary and medicinal purposes. The leaves and flowers can also be used in specific preparations.

**Components:**
Ginger contains active compounds such as gingerol, shogaol and zingiberene, which give it medicinal properties. It also contains antioxidants, vitamins and minerals.

Ginger is a perennial plant native to tropical Asia. Due to its multiple health benefits, it has been used for centuries as a spice in cooking and traditional medicine.

**History and tradition:**
This plant has been cultivated and used in Asia for over 5,000 years. It is believed to have originated in the coastal regions of South Asia, specifically in what is today known as India and China. From there, it spread to various parts of the world and was integrated into the culinary and medicinal traditions of many cultures.

Ginger is especially valued in traditional Asian medicine, such as Ayurvedic and Chinese medicine. In these traditions, it is considered a "hot" plant that can help balance the body and treat various ailments. It has been used to relieve digestive issues, including nausea, vomiting, and indigestion. In addition, it has been used as a general tonic to strengthen the immune system and promote blood circulation.

**Therapeutic properties:**
Ginger contains bioactive compounds, including gingerols and shogaols, which lend it its medicinal properties. These compounds are responsible for ginger's characteristic flavor and aroma, and they also offer numerous health benefits to the human body.

One of ginger's best-known properties is its ability to relieve nausea and vomiting. Numerous studies have shown that ginger consumption can effectively relieve nausea caused by pregnancy, chemotherapy, or surgery. The compounds in ginger act on the digestive system, reducing discomfort and improving intestinal motility.

Additionally, ginger has been used to relieve pain and inflammation. Gingerols and shogaols have been shown to have anti-inflammatory and analgesic properties, making them a natural choice for pain relief in conditions such as arthritis, muscle aches and migraines. Some studies even suggest that regular consumption of ginger may help reduce chronic inflammation in the body.

Ginger may also have positive effects on cardiovascular health. Regular consumption of ginger has been suggested to help reduce cholesterol and triglyceride levels in the blood, as well as improve blood circulation. These effects could contribute to heart health and reduce the risk of cardiovascular disease.

In addition to its therapeutic properties, ginger is also used as a spice in cooking due to its spicy and aromatic flavor. It is added to savory and sweet dishes, as well as to beverages such as ginger tea. Its culinary versatility makes it popular in many cultures and cuisines worldwide.

### Curiosities:
Ginger, whose scientific name is Zingiber officinale, is a plant native to tropical Asia. It has been used for centuries in cooking and traditional medicine due to its medicinal properties. Here are some interesting facts about ginger:

Spicy and refreshing flavor: Ginger has a distinctive taste and a refreshing touch. This characteristic flavor is attributed to active compounds such as gingerols and shogaols, which also contribute to its medicinal properties.

Ancient use: Ginger has been used in traditional Chinese and Indian medicine for over 2,000 years to treat a range of conditions, including digestive problems, muscle aches, and colds.

Culinary use: Ginger is a trendy cooking spice. Besides its medicinal properties, it is used in sweet and savory dishes, such as curries, desserts, infusions, and refreshing drinks like ginger ale.

### Adverse or side effects:
Although ginger is generally safe for most people when consumed in moderate amounts, some people may experience adverse side effects:

Upset stomach: Excessive consumption of ginger may cause an upset stomach, nausea, heartburn, or diarrhea in some people. These side effects are usually mild and go away on their own.

Interactions with medications: It may interact with certain medications, including anticoagulants and antihypertensive drugs. When combining ginger with these medications, caution is advised; it is essential to consult a physician.

Allergic reactions: Although rare, some people may be allergic to ginger. These reactions may manifest as skin rashes, itching, swelling, or difficulty breathing. If you experience any allergic reactions, seek medical attention immediately.

**Contraindications:**
There are contraindications to take into account when using ginger:

Coagulation disorders: Because ginger can inhibit platelet aggregation, caution should be exercised in people with coagulation disorders or who take anticoagulant drugs. A physician should be consulted before use.

Pregnancy and lactation: Although ginger has traditionally been used to alleviate morning sickness, it should be used with caution during pregnancy and lactation. A physician should be consulted before using it during these stages.

**Interactions:**
It can interact with certain medications and supplements, so it is essential to use caution when combining it with other treatments. Some known interactions include:

Anticoagulants: Ginger, which inhibits platelet aggregation, may increase the risk of bleeding when taken in combination with anticoagulant medications, such as warfarin. Medical supervision is recommended if both treatments are used.

Antihypertensives: Ginger may have hypotensive effects, which could interact with high blood pressure medications. If you are taking medicines for hypertension, exercise caution and consult a physician before using ginger.

# Licorice (Glycyrrhiza glabra)

**Description:**
Licorice is a perennial plant in the legume family. Its erect and branched stem can reach a height of up to 1 meter. Its leaves are pinnate, with elongated leaflets and a bright green color. Licorice flowers are small and violet or pale blue, grouped in clusters. The most used part of the plant is its root, which is

thick, fibrous, and dark brown.

### Habitat and cultivation:

Licorice is native to the warm, temperate regions of Europe and Asia, but it is now cultivated in various parts of the world. It prefers well-drained, fertile soils and can grow in sunny and semi-shaded areas. The plant requires a climate with moderate temperatures and sufficient water for optimal growth and development. Licorice can be propagated by seed or by dividing the roots.

### Parts used:

The most commonly used part of the licorice plant is its root, which contains most of its beneficial components. Although rare, the leaves and stems can also be used to a lesser extent. The root is harvested when the plant is at least three years old, usually in autumn, and dried for later use.

### Components:

Licorice root contains a variety of health-promoting components. One of the main components is glycyrrhizin, a compound that gives it its characteristic sweet taste. It also contains flavonoids, saponins, coumarins, essential oils and phytosterols. These compounds have antioxidant, anti-inflammatory, antimicrobial, and antiviral properties.

### History and tradition:

Licorice has a long history of use in traditional medicine in various cultures. It is believed to have been first used in ancient Mesopotamia more than 4,000 years ago. The Egyptians, Greeks and Romans all valued licorice for its medicinal properties and sweet taste. In traditional Chinese medicine, licorice has been used for centuries as a tonic for the respiratory and digestive systems. Due to its sweet and characteristic flavor, licorice has also been used to manufacture candies, sweets and confectionery products.

### Therapeutic properties:

Licorice possesses numerous therapeutic properties, making it a valuable component in natural medicine. It is primarily used as an anti-inflammatory, expectorant, and digestive aid. Due to its expectorant and lung-soothing properties, it has been used to relieve respiratory conditions, including colds, coughs, bronchitis, and asthma. It also helps alleviate digestive problems such as heartburn, indigestion, ulcers, and spasms. Additionally, licorice has been traditionally used as a tonic for the liver, kidneys, and adrenal glands. However, it is essential to note that, due to its glycyrrhizin content, excessive and prolonged consumption of licorice may have adverse effects, especially in people with certain health conditions, such as hypertension or kidney failure. Therefore, it is advisable to use licorice with caution and under the supervision of a health professional.

### Curiosities:

Licorice, scientifically known as Glycyrrhiza glabra, is a perennial plant used for various historical purposes. An exciting curiosity about licorice is its scientific name, Glycyrrhiza, which originates from the Greek and means "sweet root." This is because licorice root has a sweet taste and has traditionally been used as a natural sweetener in various culinary preparations and medicinal products. In addition, licorice has also been used in the manufacture of tobacco products, such as cigarettes and chewing gum.

### Adverse or side effects:

Although licorice is considered safe when consumed in moderate amounts, excessive consumption may have adverse effects. One of the main components of licorice is glycyrrhizin, which can cause fluid retention and raise blood pressure in some people. This can be especially worrisome for those who already suffer from hypertension or heart problems. Additionally, prolonged and excessive consumption of licorice can lead to electrolyte imbalances, including decreased potassium levels in the body. Cases of kidney and hormone damage have also been reported in people who have consumed large amounts of licorice over prolonged periods.

### Contraindications:

Licorice has some crucial contraindications that need to be taken into account. Its consumption is not recommended for pregnant women since glycyrrhizin can cross the placenta and affect the fetus. It is also not recommended during breast-feeding, as some components of licorice can pass into breast milk. In addition, people suffering from hypertension, heart disease, kidney failure, hormonal disorders, or diabetes should avoid or limit consumption of licorice due to possible adverse effects.

**Interactions:**
Licorice may interact with certain medications and herbs, enhancing or diminishing their effect. For example, consumption of licorice may increase the effects of medicines used to treat hypertension, which can lead to a dangerous drop in blood pressure. It may also interact with blood-thinning medications, such as warfarin, and increase the risk of bleeding. In addition, licorice may interfere with some medicines used to treat diabetes, as it can affect blood sugar levels. Therefore, it is essential to consult a healthcare professional before combining licorice with other medications or herbs to prevent potential interactions.

# Mallow (Malva sylvestris)

**Description:**
Mallow or Malva sylvestris is a perennial herbaceous plant in the Malvaceae family. Its erect, branched stem can reach a height of up to 1 meter. The leaves are large, palmate, and toothed, with a bright green color. The funnel-shaped flowers vary in color from pale pink to deep purple. This plant is known for its beauty and is used in ornamental gardens and traditional medicine.

**Habitat and cultivation:**
Mallow is native to Europe and is commonly found in meadows, along roadsides, and in wastelands. It adapts to different types of soils, although it prefers well-drained, nutrient-rich soils. This plant can grow in temperate and warm climates, tolerating direct sun and partial shade. Mallow is easily propagated by seed and can also be grown from cuttings.

**Parts used:**

Mallow leaves and flowers are mainly used for medicinal purposes. The leaves are harvested when the plant is fully mature, while the flowers are harvested when they are fully open and in bloom. The dried parts of the plant are then used to prepare infusions, extracts, or ointments.

**Components:**
Mallow contains several bioactive compounds that contribute to its therapeutic properties. These include mucilages, gel-like substances with emollient and softening properties. It also contains flavonoids, antioxidants and phenolic compounds, which may have anti-inflammatory and antioxidant effects.

**History and tradition:**
Mallow has been used in traditional medicine for centuries. The ancient Egyptians and Greeks, for example, are believed to have used it to treat various conditions, including respiratory diseases, skin irritations, and digestive disorders. Additionally, in some traditions, it is considered a sacred plant due to its protective and magical properties.

**Therapeutic properties:**
Mallow is used in herbal medicine because of its therapeutic properties. It is attributed with anti-inflammatory, emollient, soothing, and healing properties. Therefore, it treats respiratory conditions, such as coughs and colds, as well as digestive problems, including gastritis and heartburn. It is also used topically to relieve skin irritation such as minor burns, rashes and insect bites.

**Curiosities:**
Mallow, also known as Malva sylvestris, is an herbaceous perennial plant with exciting curiosities. For example, it has been used since ancient times for its medicinal properties and was attributed with magical and protective properties. In addition, this plant is known for its beauty, as it produces showy flowers in shades ranging from light pink to deep purple.

**Adverse or side effects:**
Although mallow is generally considered safe, adverse or side effects may occur in rare cases. Some people may experience

allergic reactions when they come into contact with the plant or consume its parts. Additionally, excessive consumption of mallow may have a laxative effect, causing diarrhea. It is important to note that, as with any medicinal plant, it is advisable to use it in moderation and consult a health professional if adverse effects occur.

### Contraindications:
Mallow has no significant contraindications; however, caution is advised in certain instances. For example, people with a history of allergies or sensitivity to other plants in the Malvaceae family may be at increased risk of allergic reactions to mallow. Additionally, it is recommended to avoid using mallow during pregnancy and lactation, as there have been insufficient studies to determine its safety in these stages of life.

### Interactions:
Mallow has not been associated with significant drug or supplement interactions. However, it is always advisable to consult a healthcare professional if you are taking any medications or have pre-existing health conditions before using Mallow therapeutically. This is especially relevant if you take anticoagulants or other drugs that may interact with herbs or medicinal plants.

# Marshmallow Root (Althaea officinalis)

### Description:
Marshmallow root is a perennial herbaceous plant of the Malvaceae family. Its erect, hairy stem can reach a height of up to 1.5 meters. The leaves are large, lobed, and toothed, and dark green. The marshmallow flowers are large and showy, with five petals in shades ranging from white to light pink or purple. The plant has a thick, fleshy taproot used for medicinal purposes.

### Habitat and cultivation:
Marshmallow root is native to Europe and grows in moist areas such as riverbanks and ponds. It prefers nutrient-rich, well-drained soils and is cold-hardy but can grow in warmer

climates. Marshmallows can be propagated through seed or root division. It is a hardy plant and easy to grow in gardens and orchards.

### Parts used:

Marshmallow root is the most commonly used medicinally. It is harvested in autumn when the plant has completed its growth cycle and the leaves have fallen. The root is dried and used to prepare infusions, extracts and ointments. The leaves and flowers can also be used, although to a lesser extent.

### Components:

Marshmallow root contains several active components that give it its medicinal properties. Among them are mucilages and gelatinous substances that are emollient and softening. It also contains flavonoids, tannins, phenolic acids, and allantoin, which may have anti-inflammatory, antioxidant, and healing properties.

### History and tradition:

Marshmallow root has been used for medicinal and culinary purposes since ancient times. The Egyptians and Greeks used it to treat respiratory, digestive, and skin conditions. In popular tradition, Marshmallows are believed to have protective properties and ward off evil spirits. They are also attributed to aphrodisiac properties and have been used in rituals related to love and fertility.

### Therapeutic properties:

This plant is used in herbal medicine due to its therapeutic properties. It is attributed with anti-inflammatory, emollient, soothing, and healing properties. Therefore, it relieves irritation and inflammation of the throat, as well as symptoms associated with cough, cold, bronchitis, and digestive problems such as gastritis and ulcers. It is also topically used to reduce skin irritation, minor burns, insect bites, and wounds.

### Curiosities:

Marshmallow root has some exciting curiosities. For example, its scientific name, Althaea, is derived from the Greek word"cure" or "healing", reflecting its long history of medicinal use. In addition, marshmallows have traditionally been made from the plant's root, resulting in soft, sticky candies. These candies were named after the marshmallow because of their smooth, sticky texture.

### Adverse or side effects:
Although it is generally considered safe, adverse or side effects may occur in rare cases. Some people may experience allergic reactions when they come into contact with the plant or consume its parts. Additionally, excessive marshmallow consumption may have a laxative effect, leading to diarrhea. It is important to note that, as with any medicinal plant, it is advisable to use it in moderation and consult a health professional if adverse effects occur.

### Contraindications:
There are no significant contraindications; however, caution is advised in certain instances. For example, people with a history of allergies or sensitivity to other plants in the Malvaceae family may be at increased risk of allergic reactions to Marshmallow. Additionally, it is recommended to avoid using marshmallows during pregnancy and breastfeeding, as there have been insufficient studies conducted to determine their safety in these stages of life.

### Interactions:
Marshmallow root has not been associated with significant drug or supplement interactions. However, it is always advisable to consult a healthcare professional if you are taking any medications or have pre-existing health conditions before using Marshmallow therapeutically. This is especially relevant if you take anticoagulants or other drugs that may interact with herbs or medicinal plants.

# Peppermint (Mentha)

### Description:
Peppermint or mint, scientifically known as Mentha, is a genus of herbaceous perennial plants of the Lamiaceae family.

There are many varieties of mint, but they are generally characterized by square stems, opposite leaves, and small flowers grouped in inflorescences.

**Habitat and cultivation:**
Mint is a plant found mainly in temperate regions, although some species can adapt to warmer climates. It prefers moist, fertile soils and grows best in good sun exposure or partial shade. Mint is easily grown in gardens and pots and is propagated by cuttings or root division.

**Parts used:**
Both leaves and flowers are used for medicinal and culinary purposes. The leaves are typically more aromatic and are used either fresh or dried to make infusions, teas, condiments, and essential oils. The flowers are also used, although to a lesser extent, in preparing infusions and as a decorative element in culinary dishes.

**Components:**
Peppermint contains various chemical compounds that give it its aromatic and therapeutic properties. These include menthol, menthone, limonene, carvone and cineol, among other volatile compounds. Additionally, it contains flavonoids, antioxidants, and phenolic acids, which contribute to its medicinal properties.

**History and tradition:**
Various cultures around the world have used mint since ancient times. Its medicinal use dates back to ancient Greece and Rome, where it was used to treat digestive and respiratory problems. Mint was also used in religious rituals and as an ornament in wreaths and garlands. It has been prized for its refreshing aroma and healing properties throughout history.

**Therapeutic properties:**
It has several therapeutic properties that make it valuable in traditional and alternative medicine. Its benefits include:

‣ Relief of digestive problems such as indigestion, nausea and abdominal pain.

‣ It is soothing for headaches and migraines.
‣ Decongestant and expectorant in cases of colds and nasal congestion.
‣ Antimicrobial and anti-inflammatory properties.
‣ Stimulation of digestion and increased appetite.
‣ Relaxing effect and relief of stress and anxiety.

**Curiosities:**
Peppermint is widely known for its refreshing aroma and distinctive flavor. It is used in various products, including candies, chewing gum, sweets, and oral care products.

There are many varieties of mint, including spearmint, peppermint, apple mint, and chocolate mint, each with its distinctive aroma and flavor.

Mint has been used since ancient times for its medicinal properties, as an ornamental plant, and as a natural insect repellent.

Some mint species, such as peppermint, contain high concentrations of menthol, which gives them a cooling and soothing effect.

Peppermint has traditionally been used in herbal medicine to treat digestive problems, headaches, cold symptoms and nasal congestion.

**Adverse or side effects:**
In general, peppermint is safe and well-tolerated by most people when consumed in moderate amounts as part of the diet.

However, in very high doses or sensitive people, peppermint may cause adverse effects such as heartburn, sour stomach, gastrointestinal tract irritation, or acid reflux.

Some people may experience allergies to peppermint, which may cause symptoms such as rashes, itching, swelling, or difficulty breathing.

When applied directly to the skin in high concentrations, peppermint essential oil may cause skin irritation or sensitivity in some people.

**Contraindications:**
Although it is generally safe, there are some contraindications to be aware of:

People suffering from gastroesophageal diseases such as gastroesophageal reflux disease (GERD) or peptic ulcer may experience worsening symptoms if they consume peppermint due to its relaxing effect on the lower esophageal sphincter.

People with gallbladder disorders should also use caution, as peppermint may stimulate bile production and trigger symptoms in some cases.

In rare cases, peppermint may cause irritable bowel syndrome (IBS) in susceptible people.

**Interactions:**
Peppermint may interact with certain medications; therefore, it is essential to exercise caution and consult a healthcare professional if you are taking specific medications.

The menthol present in peppermint may increase the absorption of certain drugs, potentially leading to higher levels of these drugs in the body.

Some medications that may interact with peppermint include calcium channel blockers, proton pump inhibitors (PPIs), and anticoagulants.


# **Plantain** (Plantago major)


**Description:**
It is a plant that usually grows in grassland areas, meadows and roadsides. It has a distinctive appearance, characterized by rosette-shaped basal leaves that are oval and toothed along the

edges. The leaves are deep green and can grow to approximately 20 centimeters in length. As for its flowering, plantain produces spikes of small, white flowers that rise above the foliage.

### Habitat and cultivation:

Plantain is native to Europe but has naturalized in many other regions, including North America. It is a hardy plant that can thrive in a wide range of soils and climatic conditions. It is commonly found in moist soils, such as meadows, gardens and cultivated fields. In terms of cultivation, plantain can be easily propagated from seed or by dividing the roots of mature plants.

### Parts used:

Plantain's medicinal parts are mainly its leaves and seeds. The leaves are harvested when the plant is fully grown and dried for later use. The seeds can also be collected and used fresh or dried.

### Components:

It contains a variety of active components that give it its medicinal properties. Among these components are mucilages, which are gelatinous substances that help soothe irritation and protect mucous membranes. It also contains tannins, salicylic acid, flavonoids, and triterpenoids, contributing to its therapeutic effects.

### History and tradition:

Plantain has a long history of medicinal use, dating back to antiquity. Records of its use have been found in the traditional medicine of several cultures, including those of the Greeks, Romans, and Chinese. In Europe, plantain was known as a "cure-all" plant due to its wide range of therapeutic applications.

### Therapeutic properties:

Scientific studies and traditional experience have supported several therapeutic properties, including its potential benefits as an anti-inflammatory, antioxidant, antiviral, and antibacterial agent. It has been used to treat respiratory conditions such as coughs and the common cold, relieve skin irritation, and promote wound healing. It has also been used to alleviate digestive problems, including diarrhea and gastritis.

**Curiosities:**
Plantain, or Plantago major, is a perennial herbaceous plant commonly found in temperate regions worldwide.

It has been used for centuries in traditional medicine due to its medicinal properties.

Plantain has leaves in the form of a basal rosette and has a spike-shaped inflorescence with tiny flowers.

It is a hardy plant that can grow in a wide range of soil types and climatic conditions.

Plantain is used medicinally and in cooking as an ingredient in salads and stews.

**Adverse or side effects:**
Plantain is generally considered safe for human consumption. However, some people may experience mild side effects, such as stomach upset, diarrhea, or skin allergies.

In rare cases, severe allergic reactions, such as difficulty breathing, swelling of the face or throat, and severe skin rashes, have been reported. If any of these symptoms occur, seek medical attention immediately.

**Contraindications:**
Although plantain is generally safe for most people, there are some contraindications to be aware of.

Pregnant or breastfeeding women should avoid the consumption of plantain, as there have not been enough studies on its effects on these groups.

People taking anticoagulant or antiplatelet medications should be cautious, as plantain may have anticoagulant properties and could increase the risk of bleeding.

Those with known allergies to plants of the Plantaginaceae

family should avoid plantain, as they may experience allergic reactions.

**Interactions:**
It is important to note that plantain may interact with certain medications. If you are taking any medications, it is advisable to consult a healthcare professional before using plantain supplements.

It has been reported that plantain may decrease the absorption of some oral medications, such as tricyclic antidepressants and heart medications.

Additionally, plantain may interact with immunosuppressive drugs, such as corticosteroids, and decrease their effectiveness.

If you are taking prescription medications or have a medical condition, it is essential to talk to your doctor before using plantain to avoid possible negative interactions.

# Rhubarb (Rheum rhabarbarum)

**Description:**
Rhubarb is a perennial plant in the Polygonaceae family. Its thick, fleshy stem, usually red or green, can reach a height of 1 to 2 meters. Its large, rough leaves are heart-shaped. Rhubarb flowers are small and green, grouped in a panicle-shaped inflorescence.

**Habitat and cultivation:**
It is native to the mountainous regions of Central Asia but has been cultivated in various parts of the world for its culinary and medicinal uses. It prefers cool, temperate climates with cold winters and moderate summers and grows best in nutrient-rich, well-drained soils.

**Parts used:**
The parts used are mainly the stems. The plant's leaves are not edible due to their high oxalic acid content, which can be

toxic in large quantities. Therefore, it is recommended that you avoid consuming the leaves and focus on the stems.

### Components:
Rhubarb contains several components that give it its particular characteristics. These include phenolic compounds, such as quercetin and gallic acid. It also contains malic acid, oxalic acid, and dietary fiber, which are responsible for their therapeutic properties and health benefits.

### History and tradition:
It has been used for centuries in traditional Chinese medicine, with its medicinal use believed to date back over 2,000 years. Initially, it was used primarily to promote gastrointestinal function and treat constipation. Over time, its use has been extended to other therapeutic applications.

### Therapeutic properties:
Rhubarb has traditionally been used as a natural laxative due to its compound content, including malic and oxalic acids. These compounds stimulate bowel movements and help relieve constipation. Additionally, rhubarb has been investigated for its potential antioxidant, anti-inflammatory, and antimicrobial properties. However, it is essential to note that rhubarb should be used with caution and under the supervision of a health professional, as excessive consumption can have adverse effects.

### Curiosities:
Rhubarb is widely used in cooking, especially in desserts and jams. Its stalks add a tart and slightly sweet flavor to recipes.

Although it is considered a perennial plant, it is often grown annually, as its stems are more tender when young.

Rhubarb is a hardy plant that can be grown in home gardens. However, it takes time to establish a healthy crop, and it is generally recommended not to harvest the stalks for the first two years.

### Adverse or side effects:

Excessive consumption of rhubarb may have adverse effects. Its oxalic acid content may contribute to the formation of kidney stones in susceptible people.

Additionally, consuming oxalic acid in large amounts can interfere with the absorption of certain minerals, such as calcium and iron. Therefore, moderate rhubarb consumption is recommended, especially for people with kidney problems or a history of kidney stones.

### Contraindications:
Rhubarb is contraindicated in people with intestinal obstruction, ulcerative colitis, Crohn's disease, or other inflammatory gastrointestinal disorders.

Its consumption is also discouraged during pregnancy and lactation, as there have not been enough studies to evaluate its safety in these stages.

People taking certain medications, such as anticoagulants, antihypertensives, or diuretics, should be cautious when consuming rhubarb due to possible drug-drug interactions.

### Interactions:
Rhubarb may interact with some medications. For example, the simultaneous consumption of rhubarb and some anticoagulants, such as warfarin, may increase the risk of bleeding.

There may also be interactions with diuretic and antihypertensive drugs since rhubarb has diuretic properties and may potentiate the effects of these drugs.

If you are taking any drugs, it is essential to consult with a healthcare professional before consuming rhubarb to ensure that there are no risks of interactions.

# Senna (Cassia angustifolia)

### Description:

Sen is a perennial plant in the legume family native to the tropical regions of Africa and Arabia. It reaches a height of 0.5 to 1 meter and has an erect and branched stem. Its leaves are green and lanceolate, growing in pairs that are opposite to each other. The flowers are small and pale yellow and grouped in terminal clusters. The Sen fruit is an elongated, slender pod containing brown seeds.

### Habitat and cultivation:

Sen is mainly grown in tropical and subtropical regions, such as India, Sudan, Ethiopia and Pakistan. It prefers well-drained, fertile soil and requires full sun exposure for optimal growth. Sen is propagated by seeds sown in spring. The plant requires regular but moderate watering. It is harvested when the leaves turn dark green, usually after 8 to 10 weeks of sowing.

### Parts used:

The parts of the Sen plant used for medicinal purposes are the leaves and fruit pods. The leaves are harvested and dried for later use.

### Components:

Senna contains several active components derived from anthraquinones, including sennosides A and B. These compounds are responsible for the laxative and stimulant properties of senna. In addition, the plant also contains polysaccharides, essential oils, tannins and flavonoids.

### History and tradition:

Senna's use as a medicinal plant dates back to ancient times. The ancient Egyptians are believed to have used Sen as a laxative, and there is evidence of its use in Hindu medical texts dating back over 3,000 years. It is also mentioned in traditional Arabic and Greek medicine. Over the centuries, senna has been valued for its purgative properties and used to treat constipation.

### Therapeutic properties:

Senna is mainly known for its laxative properties. The plant's sennosides stimulate intestinal contractions, accelerating intestinal transit and relieving occasional constipation. However, prolonged use or excessive doses may cause side effects such as abdominal cramps and diarrhea.

In addition to its laxative effect, Sen has also been used in traditional medicine to treat conditions such as hemorrhoids, liver problems and fever.

### Curiosities:
Senna has been used for centuries as a natural laxative and is credited with efficacy in relieving occasional constipation.

Sen has been used in religious ceremonies and purification rituals in some cultures.

Scientific research has focused on the plant due to its medicinal properties and potential as a source of bioactive compounds.

Senna is an essential plant in the pharmaceutical industry. It is an ingredient in many laxative products.

### Adverse or side effects:
Prolonged use or excessive doses of Sen can cause adverse effects, such as abdominal cramps, diarrhea, dehydration and electrolyte imbalances.

Some people may experience allergic reactions to Sen, such as rashes, itching, or swelling.

Chronic use of Sen as a laxative can lead to dependence and weakening of the intestinal muscle, which may worsen constipation in the long term.

### Contraindications:
Sen is contraindicated in people with intestinal obstruction, appendicitis, inflammatory bowel disease, severe gastro-intestinal disorders, or unexplained abdominal pain.

Pregnant or breastfeeding women should avoid the use of Sen, as there is insufficient scientific evidence on its safety during these stages.

People with chronic diseases, such as kidney disease, liver disease, diabetes, or heart disorders, should consult a physician before taking it.

### Interactions:
Sen may interact with certain drugs, such as diuretics, corticosteroids, antiarrhythmics, and medications used to treat heart disease, high blood pressure and other disorders.

It may also decrease the absorption of other drugs when taken simultaneously, which may affect their efficacy.

If you are taking any medications, consult a physician or pharmacist before using Sen to avoid potential adverse interactions.

# Spearmint (Mentha spicata)

### Description:
Spearmint is a perennial aromatic plant in the Lamiaceae family. It can grow creeping or erect and reach a height of up to 60 centimeters. Its leaves are oval, toothed, deep green, and have a characteristic fresh, minty aroma.

### Habitat and cultivation:
Spearmint is native to Europe and has spread to other parts of the world. It adapts well to different climates and soils. For optimal growth, it prefers humid, semi-shaded areas. It is an easy plant to grow and can be reproduced from seeds or by dividing its roots.

### Parts used:
The most used parts are its leaves and stems. These are harvested before the plant flowers, as their essential oil content is higher and their flavor more intense at this time.

### Components:
Spearmint contains various chemical components that are beneficial to health. Among them are essential oils, such as menthol, carvone and limonene, which give it its characteristic

aroma. It also contains flavonoids, tannins and rosmarinic acid, which have antioxidant and anti-inflammatory properties.

**History and tradition:**
Different cultures have used it since ancient times. In traditional medicine, it is attributed to stimulant, digestive, and carminative properties. It has also been used as an aromatic plant in cooking and the preparation of refreshing infusions. Historically, spearmint has been valued for its aroma and flavor, and has been used in the preparation of food, beverages, and cosmetic products.

**Therapeutic properties:**
Spearmint has several therapeutic properties. Its digestive properties help relieve symptoms of indigestion, flatulence, and nausea. Thanks to its cooling and analgesic effect, it is also used to relieve headaches and migraines. Additionally, expectorant properties help alleviate nasal congestion and coughs. The menthol in spearmint has a cooling effect and can help reduce skin irritation and itching caused by insect bites.

**Curiosities:**
Spearmint, common mint, garden mint, or lamb mint, is an aromatic plant from the Lamiaceae family.

It is commonly used in cooking to add flavor and aroma to various dishes, such as soups, salads, desserts and infusions.

Spearmint has been used since ancient times for its medicinal properties, such as relieving digestive problems, soothing headaches, and reducing stress.

It is an easy plant to grow and can be found in many regions of the world.

**Adverse or side effects:**
Although spearmint is generally safe for most people when consumed in moderate amounts, some people may experience adverse effects:

Spearmint may cause heartburn, sour stomach, or gastrointestinal irritation at high doses.

Some people may be allergic to spearmint, which can cause symptoms such as rashes, itching, swelling, or difficulty breathing.

In rare cases, spearmint may interact with certain medications, causing unwanted side effects.

**Contraindications:**
Although Spearmint is considered safe in moderate amounts, there are some contraindications to be aware of:

Pregnant women should avoid consuming large amounts of spearmint, as it can stimulate the uterus and cause contractions.

People suffering from acid reflux, stomach ulcers, or gastroesophageal reflux disease (GERD) should be cautious when consuming spearmint, as it may worsen these problems.

Those with known allergies to other plants in the Lamiaceae family, such as mint or rosemary, may be at greater risk of being allergic to Spearmint.

**Interactions:**
Spearmint can interact with certain medications, so it is essential to exercise caution when taking any medication.

It may increase the sedative effects of drugs such as barbiturates, antihistamines and medications for anxiety or insomnia.

It can also interfere with iron absorption, so separating the intake of iron supplements from spearmint is recommended.

Suppose you take specific medications, such as angiotensin-converting enzyme inhibitors (ACE inhibitors) or calcium channel blockers. In that case, it is advisable to consult your doctor before consuming spearmint, as there may be interactions.

# FINAL NOTE

Thank you very much for choosing this book to accompany you on your path to complete health. If you find the information, advice, or remedies I share here useful, would you do me a favor? Taking a moment to leave your review or rating (several stars would be greatly appreciated) is an incredible way to help me continue creating valuable content while also guiding others who, like you, are seeking to improve their health and well-being. Thank you so much for being part of this wellness community!

With gratitude,

Isabel

**Important Note on Printing and Shipping:**
All of my paperback books are printed and distributed exclusively by Amazon and its affiliated printing facilities. If you encounter any issues with print quality or delivery, please contact Amazon Customer Service directly for assistance.

As the author, I have no control over these processes, so I kindly request that your reviews focus solely on the content, remedies, or information within this work. Some readers leave negative ratings due to shipping or binding issues, unaware that these matters are, unfortunately, entirely beyond my control and ability to resolve. Thank you from the bottom of my heart for your understanding!

# AUTHOR'S BOOKS

- **ACID REFLUX**. Foods, Supplements & Medicinal Plants
- **ALLERGIES**. Foods, Supplements & Herbs
- **ANXIETY**. Foods, Supplements & Herbs
- **ARTHRITIS**. Foods, Supplements & Medicinal Plants
- **CHOLESTEROL**. Foods, Supplements & Medicinal Plants
- **DIABETES**. Foods, Supplements & Herbs
- **CONSTIPATION**. Foods, Supplements & Herbs
- **FIBROMYALGIA**. Foods, Supplements & Medicinal Plants
- **GASTRITIS**. Foods, Supplements & Herbs
- **HEMORRHOIDS**. Foods, Supplements & Herbs
- **HYPERTENSION**. Foods, Supplements & Medicinal Plants
- **INSOMNIA**. Foods, Supplements & Herbs
- **MENOPAUSE**. Foods, Supplements & Medicinal Plants
- **OSTEOARTHRITIS**. Foods, Supplements & Herbs
- **SIBO**. Foods, Supplements & Medicinal Plants
- **VARICOSE VEINS**. Foods, Supplements & Herbs

# Roots that Inspire: From Obstacles to New Horizons

Born in 1971 in Gáldar, Gran Canaria, Isabel grew up in an environment steeped in tradition and ancestral wisdom. Surrounded by the knowledge of her homeland, she learned from an early age to appreciate the healing power of medicinal plants, home remedies, and the importance of nutrition as foundations for nurturing both body and soul. This heritage, passed down through generations, shaped her childhood and sparked a deep passion for natural medicine–a passion that would eventually become the guiding force of her life.

The journey, however, was not without obstacles. In her youth, Isabel faced a period of profound difficulty: after her separation, she embraced the sole responsibility of raising her daughters. These were challenging times, with motherhood pushing her to her limits while simultaneously fueling her determination to persevere. Even during moments of uncertainty, she remained steadfast, drawing strength from her unwavering commitment to her values and her profound connection to natural health, which always served as her refuge and inspiration.

Rather than yielding to adversity, Isabel channeled it into a drive for learning and growth. She dedicated countless hours to studying books on medicinal plants, exploring new healing methods, and deepening her knowledge of natural remedies. Over the years, she pursued extensive training in naturopathy, nutrition, and complementary therapies, often sacrificing personal comforts to follow her passion. Her dedication not only provided for her family but also enabled her to profoundly impact the lives of those who sought her guidance. People came to trust her wisdom, turning to her for advice and support, and her efforts ignited transformations in countless lives.

A pivotal moment came in the 1990s when she made the decision to professionalize her calling. She embarked on formal training as a naturopath and therapist specializing in alternative health practices. This step was transformative, opening new doors and broadening her ability to serve others. Her expertise, combined with her authentic desire to help, allowed her to support a growing community of people. Every story of healing and recovery deepened her sense of purpose, and she rebuilt her life around her mission to uplift others.

But Isabel's hunger for knowledge and her desire to inspire others extended beyond her immediate community. In 2017, she took a bold new step: she began to write with the aim of sharing her hard-earned experiences and knowledge on a larger scale. Her books, written in an accessible and heartfelt style, are both informative and empowering. They seamlessly blend practical advice, recipes, and natural health alternatives, inspiring readers to embrace healthier, more balanced lifestyles. Every page radiates her warmth and passion, inviting readers to find solutions for their well-being from within and aligning them to the wisdom of nature.

Today, Isabel's work resonates with countless individuals, especially those seeking to regain their health or reconnect with a more intentional way of living. Her story stands as a powerful reminder that even the greatest challenges can lead to profound purpose. Through resilience and perseverance, she has not only transformed her own life but also paved the way for others to rediscover their harmony with nature and with themselves. Her legacy serves as a celebration of living in balance with the natural world and honoring the deep, inherent connection between humanity and the Earth—a testament that obstacles can be the stepping stones to new horizons and an invitation to care for our body, mind, and planet with respect, awareness, and love.

# BIBLIOGRAPHY & SCIENTIFIC STUDIES


1. "El poder curativo de las plantas" - Michael Castleman
2. "Plantas medicinales: El Dioscórides renovado" - Pío Font Quer
3. "The Encyclopedia of Medicinal Plants" - Andrew Chevallier
4. "Natural Health Bible for Women" - Marilyn Glenville
5. "La farmacia natural: Guía de remedios caseros a base de plantas" - James A. Duke
6. "Herbal Medicine: Biomolecular and Clinical Aspects" - Iris F. F. Benzie y Sissi Wachtel-Galor
7. "The Green Pharmacy" - James A. Duke
8. "Plantas medicinales para el estreñimiento" - Editorial Susaeta
9. "Plantas medicinales: su uso en la salud y la enfermedad" - Roberto Cáceres
10. "The Herbal Drugstore" - Linda B. White and Steven Foster
11. "The Complete Illustrated Book of Herbs" - Reader's Digest
12. "Guía de remedios naturales" - C. Norman Shealy
13. "The Complete Medicinal Herbal" - Penelope Ody
14. "Remedios herbales: Guía práctica para aliviar más de 100 dolencias comunes" - Andrew Chevallier
15. "The Essential Guide to Herbal Safety" - Simon Y. Mills y Kerry Bone
16. "Healing with Medicinal Plants of the West" - Cecilia Garcia y James D. Adams


## SCIENTIFIC STUDIES


1. "Castor oil: A vital drug for centuries" - Verma, P. R. P., & Joharapurkar, A. A.

2. "Pharmacological and therapeutic significance of Ricinus communis L". - Ogunniyi, D. S.

3. "Castor oil: An age-old therapy" - Vieira, R. D., & Simon, J. E.

4. "Magnesium carbonate and gastrointestinal health" - Schuette, S. A.

5. "Efficacy of magnesium oxide for bowel dysfunction" -

Forootan, M., Bagheri, N., & Darvishi, M.

6. "Magnesium salts in bowel preparation: A review" - Hookey, L. C., & Vanner, S. J.

7. "Nutritional and functional properties of chia seeds" - Ullah, R., Nadeem, M., & Khalique, A.

8. "Chia seed supplementation and bowel regulation" - Vuksan, V., Jenkins, A. L., & Brissette, C.

9. "Chia seeds: Historical and nutritional significance" - Reyes-Caudillo, E., Tecante, A., & Valdivia-López, M. Á.

10. "Psyllium: A dietary fiber with diverse health benefits" - Marlett, J. A., & Fischer, M. H.

11. "Psyllium fiber and bowel function: A review" - McRorie, J. W., & Fahey, G. C.

12. "The role of psyllium in constipation and health" - Anderson, J. W., & Allgood, L. D.

13. "Probiotics in the management of constipation" - Dimidi, E., Christodoulides, S., & Scott, S. M.

14. "Probiotics for functional constipation: A systematic review" - Ford, A. C., Quigley, E. M. M., & Lacy, B. E.

15. "The role of probiotics in gastrointestinal health" - Marteau, P., & Shanahan, F.

16. "Rhubarb extract in constipation: Traditional use and modern science" - Xiong, H., & Ye, X. Y.

17. "Phytochemical and pharmacological properties of rhubarb" - Guo, Y. J., & Chen, X. J.

18. "Rhubarb as a medicinal plant: Therapeutic effects on constipation" - Wang, Q., & Zhang, Y. N.

19. "Chicory root fiber and its health benefits" - Roberfroid, M. B.

20. "Chicory: A review of its traditional uses and pharmacological properties" - Street, R. A., & Sidana, J.

21. "Chicory root fiber supplementation and digestive health" - Causey, J. L., & Feirtag, J. M.

22. "Boldo: Traditional use and modern pharmacology" - Rubiolo, J. A., & López-Alonso, M.

23. "Phytochemical and pharmacological studies of Peumus boldus" - Speisky, H., & Cassels, B. K.

24. "Medicinal uses of boldo leaves: A review" - Alzamora, S. M., & López-Malo, A.

25. "Cascara sagrada: A review of its laxative properties" - Gardner, E. J.

26. "Pharmacognostic evaluation of Cascara sagrada" - Blumenthal, M., & Busse, W. R.

27. "Cascara sagrada and its use in bowel regulation" - Bradley, P. R.

28. "Dandelion: A review of its traditional uses and medicinal properties" - Yarnell, E., & Abascal, K.

29. "Dandelion root and leaf: Effects on digestive health" - Schutz, K., & Carle, R.

30. "Therapeutic benefits of dandelion in gastrointestinal disorders" - Choi, U. K., & Lee, O. H.

31. "Frangula bark: A review of its laxative properties" - Blumenthal, M., & Goldberg, A.

32. "Phytochemistry and pharmacology of Frangula alnus" - Mitaine-Offer, A. C., & Miyamoto, T.

33. "Frangula: Traditional uses and therapeutic properties" - Wichtl, M.

34. "Peppermint in gastrointestinal health: A review" - McKay, D. L., & Blumberg, J. B.

35. "Mentha piperita: Pharmacological properties and health benefits" - Balakrishnan, A.

36. "The therapeutic use of peppermint in gastrointestinal disorders" - Kligler, B., & Chaudhary, S.

37. "Fennel and its role in gastrointestinal health" - Badgujar, S. B., & Patel, V. V.

38. "Phytochemistry and pharmacological activities of Foeniculum vulgare" - Rather, M. A., & Dar, B. A.

39. "Fennel: A comprehensive review of its traditional and modern uses" - Singh, G., & Maurya, S.

40. "Ginger and its potential role in gastrointestinal disorders" - Ali, B. H., & Blunden, G.

41. "Pharmacological effects of ginger on gastrointestinal function" - Zadeh, J. B., & Kor, N. M.

42. "Ginger: An herbal remedy for digestive health" - Lete, I., & Allué, J.

43. "Plantain: Traditional uses and modern research" - Samuelsen, A. B.

44. "The medicinal uses of Plantago: A review" - Samuelsen, A. B.

45. "Phytochemistry and pharmacological properties of Plantago major" - Sagnia, B., & Gborbiah, D.

46. "Malva sylvestris: Traditional uses and pharmacological properties" - Barros, L., & Carvalho, A. M.

47. "The therapeutic potential of Malva sylvestris in digestive disorders" - Çalişkan, O., & Ceylan, O.

48. "Malva: A review of its medicinal properties and applications" - Özbek, H., & Uğraş, S.

49. "Marshmallow root: Traditional use and therapeutic benefits" - Kulp, K. S., & Montgomery, J. L.

50. "Phytochemical and pharmacological properties of Althaea officinalis" - Boskabady, M. H., & Javan, H.

51. "Herbal medicine: Marshmallow and its therapeutic effects" - Samavati, V., & Manoochehrizade, A.

52. "Chamomile: A herbal medicine of the past with bright future" - Srivastava, J. K., & Gupta, S.

53. "Therapeutic effects of Matricaria recutita in gastrointestinal disorders" - McKay, D. L., & Blumberg, J. B.

54. "Chamomile: An overview of its medicinal uses" - Srivastava, J. K., & Shankar, E.

55. "Peppermint oil and its therapeutic potential in gastrointestinal health" - Grigoleit, H. G., & Grigoleit, P.

56. "Mentha species: In vitro and in vivo assessments of their antioxidant activity" - Dorman, H. J. D., & Deans, S. G.

57. "Mints: A comparative study of their bioactivity and health benefits" - Lawrence, B. M.

58. "Licorice and its potential therapeutic effects in digestive health" - Asl, M. N., & Hosseinzadeh, H.

59. "Glycyrrhiza glabra (Licorice): A comprehensive review on its phytochemistry" - Fenwick, G. R., & Lutomski, J.

60. "Licorice: A traditional medicine for modern times" - Fiore, C., & Eisenhut, M.

61. "Rhubarb: Its role in traditional medicine and current research" - Xie, W., & Du, L.

62. "Therapeutic effects of Rheum species in digestive disorders" - Guo, H., & Zhang, L.

63. "Phytochemical and pharmacological properties of rhubarb" - Huang, Q., & Zhang, S.

64. "Senna: A traditional herbal medicine with modern applications" - Lemmens-Gruber, R., & Marchart, E.

65. "The pharmacological activities of Senna: A review" - Khare, C. P.

66. "Senna: A review of its traditional uses and modern applications in gastrointestinal health" - Bradley, P. R.

## FINAL NOTE


## AUTHOR'S BOOKS


## Roots that Inspire: From Obstacles to New Horizons


## BIBLIOGRAPHY & SCIENTIFIC STUDIES